Complications in Orthopaedics
Shoulder Arthroscopy

Edited by
Xavier A. Duralde, MD
Peachtree Orthopaedic Clinic
Assistant Clinical Professor of Orthopaedics
Emory University
Atlanta, Georgia

Series Editor
Peter C. Amadio, MD
Mayo Clinic
Rochester, Minnesota

Published by the
American Academy of Orthopaedic Surgeons
6300 North River Road
Rosemont, IL 60018

AAOS
American Academy of Orthopaedic Surgeons

American Academy of Orthopaedic Surgeons
6300 North River Road
Rosemont, IL 60018
1-800-626-6726

First Edition

ISBN 10: 0-89203-499-8
13: 978-0-89203-499-4

Contributors

Xavier A. Duralde, MD
Peachtree Orthopaedic Clinic
Assistant Clinical Professor of Orthopaedics
Emory University
Atlanta, Georgia

Donald P. Endrizzi, MD
Attending Surgeon
Orthopaedic Associates of Portland
Maine Medical Center
Portland, Maine

Douglas H. Murray, MD
Orthopaedic Surgeon
Peachtree Orthopaedic Clinic
Atlanta, Georgia

Contents

Preface

Shoulder arthroscopy emerged in the 1980s and has evolved from a simple diagnostic procedure to one that allows complex reconstructions formerly reserved for open surgery. The increase in the number and variety of procedures performed today compared with 20 years ago is astonishing. Surgeons today routinely perform multiple complex therapeutic interventions in the shoulder, including subacromial decompression, rotator cuff repair, and instability repair—a significant advancement from the 1980s when even diagnostic arthroscopy of the glenohumeral joint was a challenge.

The arthroscope has improved our understanding of shoulder anatomy and function by permitting observation of structures in a less invasive fashion, so patients too have benefited from the progression toward an arthroscopic approach to shoulder surgery, with a decreased risk of infection, reduced perioperative incisional pain, and less need for hospitalization. Throughout this evolution, surgeons have attempted to reproduce successful open techniques arthroscopically, and this trial and error has led, over a relatively short period, to great advances in surgical techniques and the equipment required to perform them. These advances, however, have come at a cost, and complications are as much a part of shoulder arthroscopy as they are in every other surgical field.[1]

Shoulder arthroscopy offers multiple unique challenges. As with other joints, the surgeon is working in a tight space; however, arthroscopy does not afford the normal tactile feedback of open surgery. There is also a significant learning curve to arthroscopic shoulder surgery because of the volume of different procedures normally performed by the shoulder surgeon. The arthroscopic approach, therefore, requires a specialist rather than a generalist.[2] From the moment the arthroscope enters the shoulder, the clock begins ticking, and the surgeon must be aware that the time to accomplish the procedure is limited by issues of fluid extravasation and tissue edema, which can occasionally lead to life-threatening complications. (The importance of edema control is emphasized repeatedly in this monograph because it is a factor in a wide variety of complications.) Surgeons must focus on doing what is best for each patient and avoid feeling that conversion from an arthroscopic to an open procedure represents a failure, because this may be the best treatment for that particular patient in the hands of that particular surgeon. Most open procedures of the shoulder have a proven record of success, and certainly a well-executed open surgery has a higher chance of ultimate success than a poorly performed arthroscopic procedure.

Complications can occur in shoulder surgery not only from the procedure itself but also from the setup and positioning of the patient. Arthroscopic shoulder procedures, therefore, must be carefully planned, from the type of anesthesia administered, to the type of positioning and traction used, to the instrumentation necessary for each step of the procedure. The unique anatomy of the shoulder offers another significant challenge to the surgeon in that a tourniquet cannot be used on the shoulder to control bleeding as with other joints. Special attention, therefore, must be given to bleeding control in this highly vascular area. Although sometimes perceived as relatively minor surgery by the patient, arthroscopic shoulder surgery is extremely demanding on the surgeon, stressful to the patient, and fraught with potential complications if not well planned.

The overall complication rate for arthroscopic surgery of the shoulder is elusive,[3] but has been quoted historically as ranging between 5.8% and 9.5% in published series.[4-8] The complication rate correlates directly with the type of surgery performed, with procedures of increased complexity, such as rotator cuff repair, having higher rates than simpler procedures, such as subacromial decompression.

The increased awareness of complications related to shoulder arthroscopy has led to advances in surgical techniques, from subtle modification in some instances to the abandonment of entire procedures in others (eg, staple capsulorrhaphy and thermal capsulorrhaphy) because of unacceptably high complication rates. Newer devices, such as thermal probes; metal, plastic, and bioabsorbable anchors; and pain pumps, must be monitored carefully and scientifically as well so that their efficacy can similarly be improved. The focus on complications, then, is a powerful learning tool that promotes the advancement of surgical techniques and improves patient care by helping surgeons avoid similar complications in the future.

Table 1: Reported Complications of Shoulder Arthroscopy[1,3,4,6]

General shoulder arthroscopy complications
- Bleeding
- Neurologic injuries
- Fluid extravasation
- Stiffness
- Iatrogenic tendon injury
- Instrument breakage
- Skin problems
- Portal placement problems
- Articular cartilage damage

Complications related to specific procedures

Subacromial surgery
- Inadequate resection
- Acromial fracture
- AC joint problems
  - Inadequate resection
  - Excessive resection with instability
- Heterotopic ossification
- Deltoid pull-off

Rotator cuff repair
- Hardware problems
  - Suture anchor displacement
  - Tuberosity overload with fracture
- Stiffness
- Failed repairs
- Suprascapular nerve injury

Instability repair
- Recurrence
- Hardware problems
- Complications of thermal capsulorrhaphy
  - Articular cartilage damage
  - Nerve injury
  - Capsular injury

Capsular release
- Nerve damage
- Articular damage

Any publication on complications runs the risk of turning into a list that may be of little help to the surgeon. Table 1 covers the gamut of reported complications of shoulder arthroscopy and is helpful to the reader in its breadth.

Ideally, however, publications of this sort should identify complications in the context of the settings in which they occur, instruct surgeons in methods to avoid complications, and describe treatment rationale for management once a complication has occurred. In this way, the surgeon can anticipate potential complications and undertake maneuvers to avoid them in the first place. When a complication does occur, the surgeon should be able to recognize it, identify the potential cause, and apply treatment strategies to manage it.

The format of this monograph is one of case reports, which will allow the surgeon to understand the contexts in which these complications can occur. The complications are organized in a diagnosis-related fashion based on the types of procedures performed in shoulder arthroscopy. The book begins with general complications associated with anesthesia and positioning, proceeding to complications associated with subacromial decompression and arthroscopic rotator cuff surgery, and finally to those related to arthroscopic instability surgery. In an attempt to avoid repetition of a recent AAOS publication on rotator cuff surgery,[9] several complications—specifically, postoperative infections after rotator cuff repair and stiffness following rotator cuff surgery—will not be discussed in this book. For a thorough and clear discussion of these issues, the reader is referred to that monograph.

Finally, I wish to thank the contributing authors and the AAOS publications staff for their support. Without their tireless efforts, this book would not have been possible.

Xavier A. Duralde, MD
Editor

References

1. Kuremsky MA, Connor PM, D'Alessandro DF: Complications of arthroscopic shoulder surgery, in Blaine TA (ed): *Shoulder Arthroscopy*. Rosemont, IL, American Academy of Orthopaedic Surgeons, 2006, pp 93-105.

2. Yamaguchi K, Levine WN, Marra G, Galatz LM, Klepps S, Flatow EL: Transitioning to arthroscopic rotator cuff repair: The pros and cons. *Instr Course Lect* 2003;52:81-92.

3. Bigliani LU, Flatow EL, Deliz ED: Complications of shoulder arthroscopy. *Orthop Rev* 1991;20:743-751.

4. Weber SC, Abrams JS, Nottage WM: Complications associated with arthroscopic shoulder surgery. *Arthroscopy* 2002;18(suppl 1):88-95.

5. Berjano P, González BG, Olmedo JF, Perez-Espana LA, Munilla MG: Complications in arthroscopic shoulder surgery. *Arthroscopy* 1998;14:785-788.

6. McFarland EG, O'Neill OR, Hsu CY: Complications of shoulder arthroscopy. *J South Orthop Assoc* 1997;6: 190-196.

7. Mueller D, Landsiedl F: Arthroscopy of the shoulder joint: A minimal invasive and harmless procedure? *Arthroscopy* 2000;16:425.

8. Small NC: Complications in arthroscopic surgery performed by experienced arthroscopists. *Arthroscopy* 1988;4:215-221.

9. Green A (ed): *Complications in Orthopaedics: Rotator Cuff Surgery*. Rosemont, IL, American Academy of Orthopaedic Surgeons, 2006.

Chapter 1

Bleeding Problems During Shoulder Arthroscopy

Xavier A. Duralde, MD

Case Presentation

A 52-year-old man is scheduled for arthroscopic subacromial decompression and rotator cuff repair of the right shoulder after a course of nonsurgical treatment fails. The patient is 6 ft tall and weighs 240 lb. MRI scans show a medium-sized, full-thickness rotator cuff tear involving the supraspinatus insertion (**Figure 1**).

Anesthetic plans include an interscalene block plus general anesthesia delivered via a laryngeal mask airway. The interscalene block was placed preoperatively in the preanesthesia holding area, and a nerve stimulator was used. Only a triceps reflex was obtained, and 30 mL of 0.5% plain bupivacaine was injected. The patient reported some numbness in his shoulder but could still elevate the arm off of the stretcher.

Initial Surgery

The surgery was performed with the patient in the beach chair position with a neurosurgical headrest. Vital signs initially were a heart rate of 60 beats/min and a blood pressure of 105/50 mm Hg. Irrigation pressure was obtained by gravity using bags of saline solution placed at 6 ft in height. No pump was used. Epinephrine was infiltrated into the first four 3-L saline bags, and 10 mL of 1:1,000 epinephrine solution (1 mg/mL) was placed into each bag for a final concentration of 1:30,000 dilution of epinephrine, or 3.3 mg/L.

The glenohumeral arthroscopy was unremarkable other than the rotator cuff tear, which could be seen from the articular side. Minimal débridement of the labrum was required. The arthroscope was then redirected via the posterior portal into the subacromial space, with fluid inflow through the cannula. The subacromial space was difficult to see because of dense bursal scarring (**Figure 2**). A midlateral portal was then established, and a 5.5-mm full-radius resector was inserted blindly into the subacromial space. The surgeon began shaving in an attempt to clear the bursa enough to expose the subacromial space and see the instrument.

The anesthesiologist reported an increase in the patient's blood pressure just as the surgeon encountered bleeding. The patient's heart rate increased to 110 beats/min and blood pressure increased to 150/90 mm Hg. The anesthesiolo-

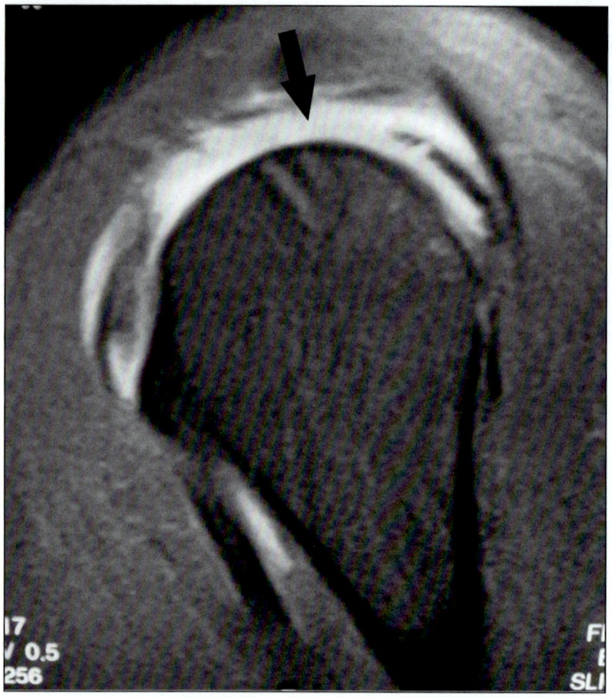

Figure 1 Sagittal oblique MRI scan of the right shoulder reveals a medium-sized rotator cuff tear primarily involving the supraspinatus tendon (arrow).

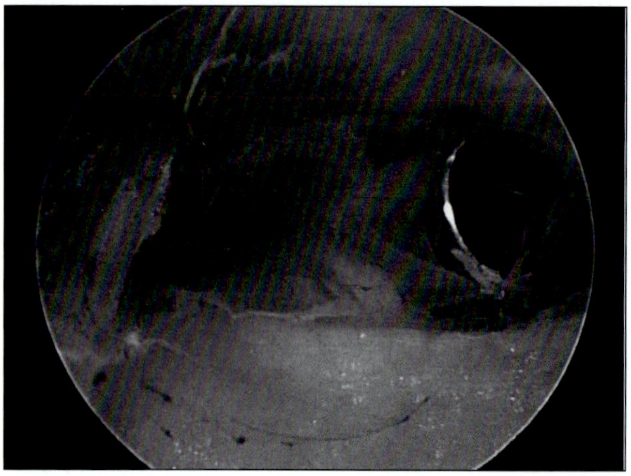

Figure 2 Dense bursal scarring in the subacromial space can limit visualization. Bursa should be cleared centrally initially to avoid bleeding vessels in the area of the AC joint.

gist increased the amount of inhalation agent to lower the blood pressure because the patient appeared to be reacting to painful stimuli. Despite

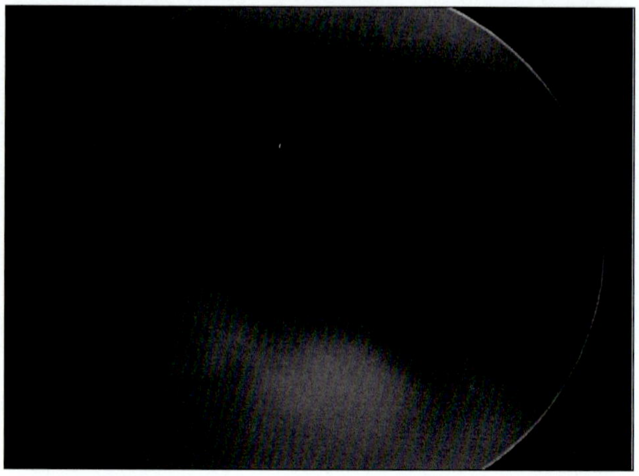

Figure 3 Bleeding in the subacromial space limits visualization and can lead to significant delays in surgery.

these measures, a "red out" occurred in the subacromial space, and visualization was extremely poor (**Figure 3**). The surgeon struggled to obtain hemostasis with an electrocautery device. Moderate shoulder edema developed, and the surgeon could not see adequately enough to continue the procedure.

Current Problem and Treatment

In this situation, inadequate hemostasis has led to total loss of visualization during arthroscopy. Sometimes, the only solution is to abort the arthroscopy and proceed with an open procedure. Many factors led to the problem, and a number of preventative maneuvers could have avoided it. Once bleeding occurs, a number of tactics can control it so that the arthroscopic procedure can proceed.

Discussion

Recognizing the Problem

Hemostasis is a unique challenge in shoulder arthroscopy because of the inability to use a tourniquet and the significant vascularity in the subacromial space. The subacromial space also is a potential space without a synovial lining, and excessive distention can lead to fluid extravasation, which can further complicate surgery. Adequate hemostasis is critical to the success of shoulder arthroscopy because this surgery cannot be performed without clear visualization. Maintaining hemostasis depends on multiple factors, including the addition of epinephrine into the irrigation fluid, a gradient in pressure between the subacromial space and the patient's systolic blood pressure, avoiding blood vessels in the subacromial space, and appropriate management of preoperative medications.

Use of Epinephrine

There is little in the orthopaedic literature concerning the ideal dilution of epinephrine in the irrigation fluid for shoulder arthroscopy. A 1:300,000 dilution of epinephrine (0.33 mg/L) in saline solution has been reported to adequately maintain hemostasis and provide visual clarity without a resultant hypertension.[1] Use of this solution has been shown to be superior to saline alone in providing a clear field of view in the subacromial space.[1] In the case presentation, a solution ten times stronger than this recommendation was used, and systemic absorption may have been partially responsible for the patient's hypertension and paradoxical increase in bleeding. Used in excess, epinephrine actually can increase the amount of bleeding encountered in shoulder arthroscopy.

Epinephrine-induced ventricular tachycardia also has been reported as a complication of shoulder arthroscopy, emphasizing the potential dangers of this agent.[2] I inject 1 mL of 1:1,000 epinephrine into the first four 3-L bags at the beginning of the procedure but none to additional fluid bags thereafter. This policy was instituted after a patient experienced a cardiac arrest thought to be related to epinephrine toxicity. Since then, thousands of these procedures have been done at our institution without problems related to intraoperative bleeding and loss of visualization. Injecting portals with an epinephrine-containing anesthetic solution may also be beneficial to limit bleeding.

Controlling Bleeding

Several anesthetic maneuvers may be beneficial in controlling intraoperative bleeding. Morrison and associates[3] reported that a pressure gradient of at least 49 mm Hg between the systolic blood pressure and subacromial space pressure is necessary to prevent bleeding from the small capillaries in that space. Hypotensive anesthesia allows for use of less pressure in the subacromial space, thereby limiting fluid extravasation and edema. Interscalene block anesthesia results in venous dilation and increases venous capacitance, which also may help limit bleeding.[4] The anesthesia provided by the interscalene block decreases afferent pain sensations and helps keep systolic blood pressure low. In the case presentation, an incomplete interscalene block may have contributed to bleeding.

Maintaining Adequate Hydrostatic Pressure

Both gravity flow and pressure pumps have been used effectively to maintain adequate hydrostatic pressure in the shoulder during arthroscopy. When gravity is used, 3-L bags of saline solution generally are elevated to 8 ft in height (**Figure 4**). Pump pressures of 50 to 60 mm Hg generally are used for glenohumeral and subacromial arthroscopy. Adequate fluid inflow is critical to maintain joint and bursal distention and hydrostatic pressure and must match the fluid outflow created by suction shavers and burrs. Gravity flow through the arthroscopic camera cannula often will not result in sufficient pressure to allow shaving with suction. If gravity flow is used, a separate 5-mm inflow cannula allows adequate flow and maintains subacromial pressure during shaving and burring. Use of suction on the shaver or burr will temporarily decrease hydrostatic pressure and may lead to bleeding. When the subacromial space is examined following bursectomy and immediately before acromioplasty, the presence of even innocent-appearing tiny red dots may represent potential bleeders that will erupt the moment the suction on the burr is turned on (**Figure 5**). Thorough hemostasis is required before proceeding to acromioplasty.

Three specific areas in the subacromial space have a network of arteries and capillaries that must be addressed by careful dissection and use of electrocautery (**Figure 6**). Fatty tissues immediately inferior and posterior to the acromioclavicular (AC) joint are rich in blood vessels and are a common source of bleeding. Dissection in this area is best performed using a cautery/ablation probe rather than a full-

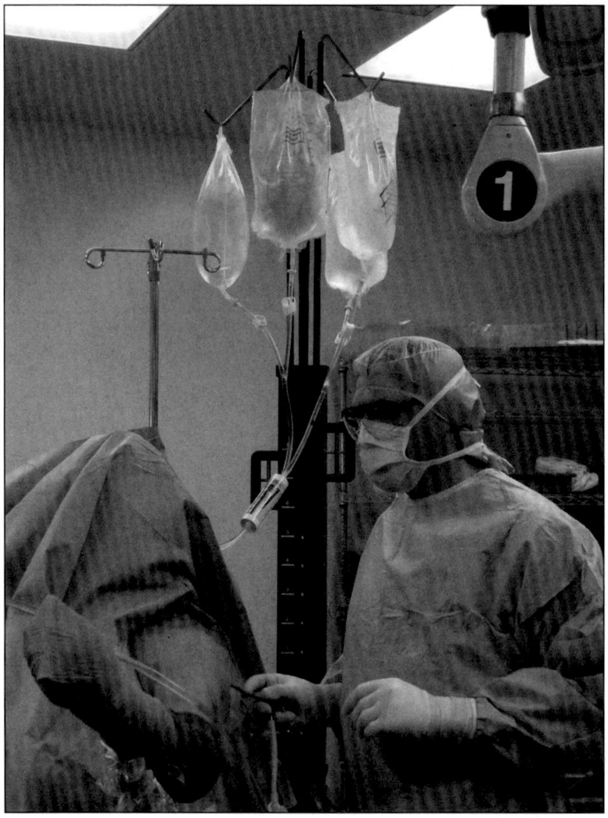

Figure 4 When using gravity inflow for shoulder arthroscopy, 3-L saline bags elevated to a height of 8 ft generally produces adequate hydrostatic pressure to ensure visualization.

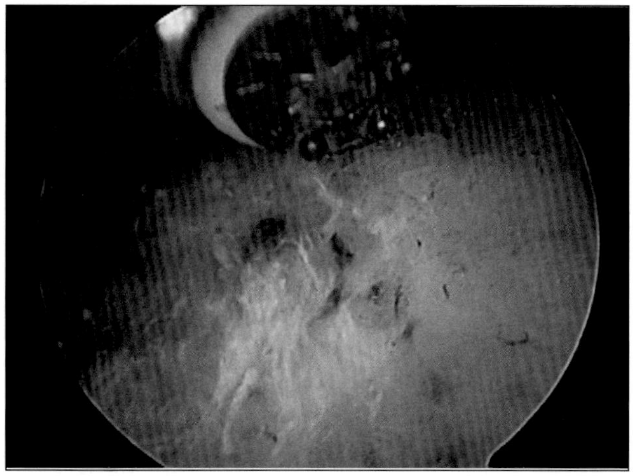

Figure 5 Innocent-appearing red dots in bursal and fatty tissue of the subacromial space can represent open vessels that will begin bleeding the moment shaving is begun and hydrostatic pressure drops. These vessels should be cauterized to avoid bleeding.

radius resector, because the ablation probe is less likely to cause bleeding and can be used to cauterize bleeding vessels simultaneously. Many of these types of probes are commercially available and are far superior to the previously used needlepoint cautery in maintaining hemostasis and safely ablating vascular tissues.

All shaving and burring should be performed under direct visualization, especially when first starting the bursectomy, because there is a tendency to insert the shaver too far medially when initially entering the subacromial space. If shaving is begun without visualizing the resector, the fatty tissue behind the AC joint may be inadvertently shaved, leading to an early and time-consuming "red out," as occurred in the case presentation. Because visualization is lost, the surgeon cannot proceed with the operation until bleeding is controlled. The time spent controlling this bleeding may be associated with increased fluid extravasation and edema, further complicating surgery. During bursectomy, the lateral gutter between the rotator cuff and deltoid can be safely shaved using a full-radius resector as long as small vessels along these structures are avoided. The shaver blade should be pointed directly posteriorly, not facing either the rotator cuff or deltoid (**Figure** 7). Resection of the bursa medially is best performed with an ablation probe to avoid bleeding.

The acromial branch of the thoracoacromial artery is encountered during takedown of the anterior portion of the coracoacromial ligament off the acromion and represents the second common site of subacromial bleeding. Carefully detaching this ligament using electrocautery rather than a shaver or burr can prevent bleeding from this vessel.

Finally, the deltoid muscle has a rich blood supply, and ablation or shaving of the muscle fibers can result in bleeding. Care should be taken to limit shaving and ablation to the bony surfaces or bursal tissues while avoiding penetration of the deltoid fascia other than for placement of cannulas.

Patients should be advised to stop taking all medications that affect coagulation, including warfarin, aspirin, and other anti-inflammatory medica-

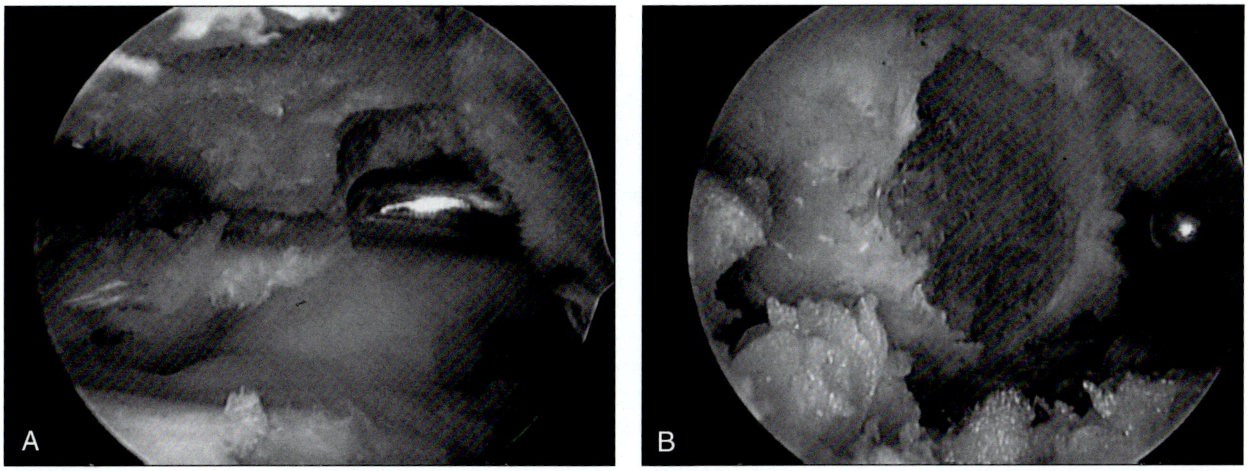

Figure 6 Three locations in subacromial arthroscopy are generally associated with bleeding and should be dealt with carefully: 1) fatty tissue adjacent to the AC joint; 2) the acromial branch of the thoracoacromial artery; and 3) the deltoid muscle. **A**, The relationship of the coracoacromial ligament and deltoid fibers to the acromion can be visualized in this arthroscopic image obtained during acromioplasty. **B**, The highly vascular fatty tissues surrounding the AC joint are clearly visualized in this photograph obtained after distal clavicle resection.

tions because these will lead to an increase in bleeding during surgery. Use of cold irrigation fluids also has been recommended to promote constriction of blood vessels, but measures should be taken to avoid hypothermia, especially with prolonged procedures that require large amounts of irrigation fluids.

Case Management and Outcome Summary

The surgeon opened the outflow from the camera to release the bloody fluid from the subacromial space. The bags with epinephrine were then removed and replaced with bags of normal saline solution without epinephrine. The bags were elevated to 8 ft in height, and the subacromial space was rinsed with normal saline solution. Bleeding vessels were identified in the fatty tissues posterior to the AC joint and adequately cauterized (**Figure** 8). The patient's blood pressure decreased to 100/50 mm Hg following administration of more inhalation agent. The subacromial pathology could then be visualized, and the arthroscopic acromioplasty, distal clavicle resection, and rotator cuff repair continued without further complication.

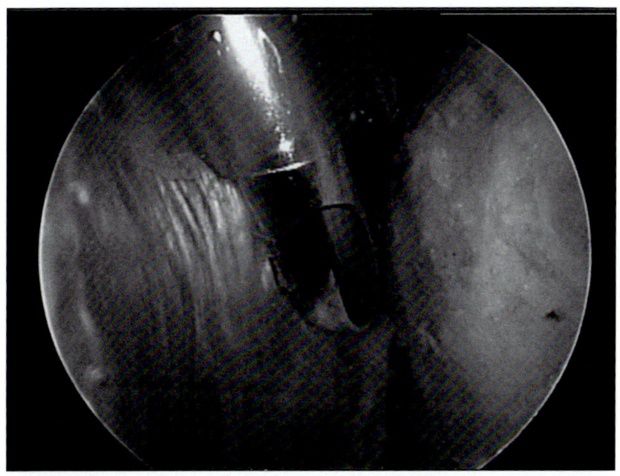

Figure 7 When clearing bursal tissue from the lateral gutter, it is critical to aim the full-radius resector away from the greater tuberosity or deltoid to avoid vessels on each of these structures.

Strategies to Minimize Common Complications

Once bleeding is encountered, a clear field of vision can be reestablished using a variety of techniques. The surgeon should move expeditiously to minimize

Table 1 Tips to Prevent Bleeding During Shoulder Arthroscopy

Goals	Strategies
Maintain adequate hydrostatic pressure gradient in the shoulder	*Hypotensive anesthesia* - Consider interscalene block *Adequate inflow* - 5-mm cannula if gravity is used - Bags of saline solution raised to 8 ft in height - Minimum pump pressure required to maintain visibility
Use electrocautery or ablation device	
Avoid bleeding vessels	- Fatty tissue adjacent to the AC joint - Acromial branch of the thoracoacromial artery - Deltoid muscle
Use of epinephrine in irrigation solution	- 0.33 mg/L of solution - 1 mL 1:1,000 epinephrine solution in each of the first four 3-L bags - No epinephrine in any additional bags

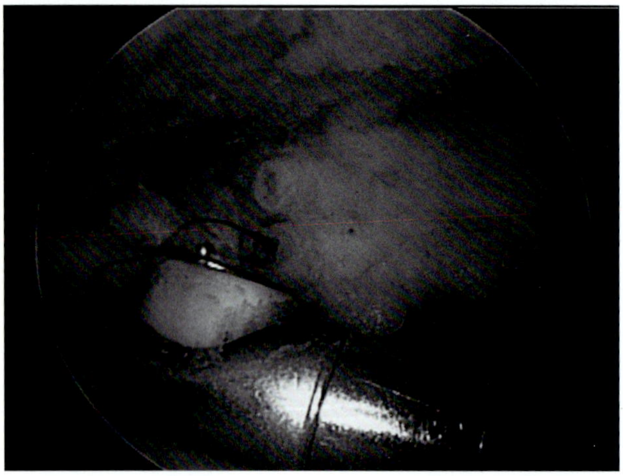

Figure 8 Fatty tissues inferior and posterior to the AC joint are rich with blood vessels and require careful cautery to avoid bleeding.

the amount of fluid extravasation and tissue edema that can occur with prolonged surgery (**Table 1**).

As mentioned previously, the pressure gradient between the systolic blood pressure and the subacromial pressure must be brought into the range of 49 mm Hg. If the patient is hypertensive, the systolic blood pressure must be lowered. Anesthetic agents can deepen the state of sedation to address issues of pain as the source of hypertension. Agents to lower the blood pressure can be given.

Epinephrine may be temporarily removed from the irrigation fluid if its absorption is thought to be associated with the increase in blood pressure. Epinephrine concentrations higher than 0.33 mg/L in irrigation fluids should be avoided. If a pump is being used, the pressure can be increased temporarily. If gravity pressure is being used, the bags can be raised. With both of these maneuvers, however, there is a risk of increased fluid extravasation and tissue edema. Therefore, these should be used as short-term solutions only. Inflow through a 5-mm cannula subacromially is preferable over inflow through the arthroscope cannula.

The surgeon should immediately focus on the most likely source of bleeding. If the coracoacromial ligament has just been released, the source of the bleeding is most likely the acromial branch of the thoracoacromial artery. If the bleeding occurs as the bursa is being shaved medially at the AC joint, the plexus of vessels surrounding this joint are the most likely source. Bleeding can originate from a location medial to the area in which the surgeon was working because the suction on the shaver can pull those tissues into the blades and then allow them to retract back to their original location.

The working cannula in the lateral portal can be maneuvered to the most likely source of bleeding and the side port opened. This allows blood to pass directly out of the cannula and avoid obscuring the subacromial space. A cautery device can then be passed down the cannula and applied to the bleeding vessel. Temporarily opening the fluid outflow on the arthroscope cannula also can help clear the water and allow visualization of the bleeding.

References

1. Jensen KH, Werther K, Stryger V, Schultz K, Falkenberg B: Arthroscopic shoulder surgery with epinephrine saline irrigation. *Arthroscopy* 2001;17:578-581.
2. Karns JL: Epinephrine-induced potentially lethal arrhythmia during arthroscopic shoulder surgery: A case report. *AANA Journal* 1999;67:419-421.
3. Morrison DS, Schaefer RK, Friedman RL: The relationship between subacromial space pressure, blood pressure, and visual clarity during arthroscopic subacromial decompression. *Arthroscopy* 1995;11:557-560.
4. Brown AR, Weiss R, Greenberg C, Flatow EL, Bigliani LU: Interscalene block for shoulder arthroscopy: Comparison with general anesthesia. *Arthroscopy* 1993;9:295-300.

Chapter 2

Severe Edema During Shoulder Arthroscopy

Xavier A. Duralde, MD

Case Presentation

A 57-year-old heavy manual laborer has chronic right shoulder impingement syndrome that has been refractory to nonsurgical management. He is 6 ft tall, weighs 260 lb, and is quite muscular. Radiographs show spur formation at the acromion and acromioclavicular joint (**Figure 1**). MRI scans show a medium-sized rotator cuff tear with retraction (**Figure 2**). He has been followed by a general orthopaedic surgeon who performs approximately 40 arthroscopic shoulder procedures per year. Because nonsurgical treatment failed, the patient was scheduled for surgery.

Initial Surgery

The surgery was performed with the patient in the lateral decubitus position under an interscalene block with sedation but without general anesthesia. The interscalene block consisted of 30 mL of 0.5% plain bupivacaine and was applied using a nerve stimulator in the preoperative holding area. Dense motor and sensory blocks were obtained, and the patient was positioned in the left lateral decubitus position on the operating table approximately 20 minutes after initiation of the block. A face shield was placed over the patient to provide an oxygen mist and to keep the surgical drapes off of his face. The patient was mildly sedated, but could communicate verbally with the anesthesiologist during the procedure. The patient was prepared and draped, and the operative arm placed in the traction device.

Upon insertion of the arthroscope into the glenohumeral joint, the surgeon noticed a tear involving approximately 50% of the thickness of the biceps tendon. The rotator cuff tear also was larger than it appeared on the MRI scan, involving the entire supraspinatus and infraspinatus tendons with retraction halfway between the greater tuberosity and glenoid (**Figure 3**). The subscapularis, however, was in good condition. As expected from preoperative radiographs, the patient had a large subacromial spur as well as spurs at the acromioclavicular joint (**Figure 4**).

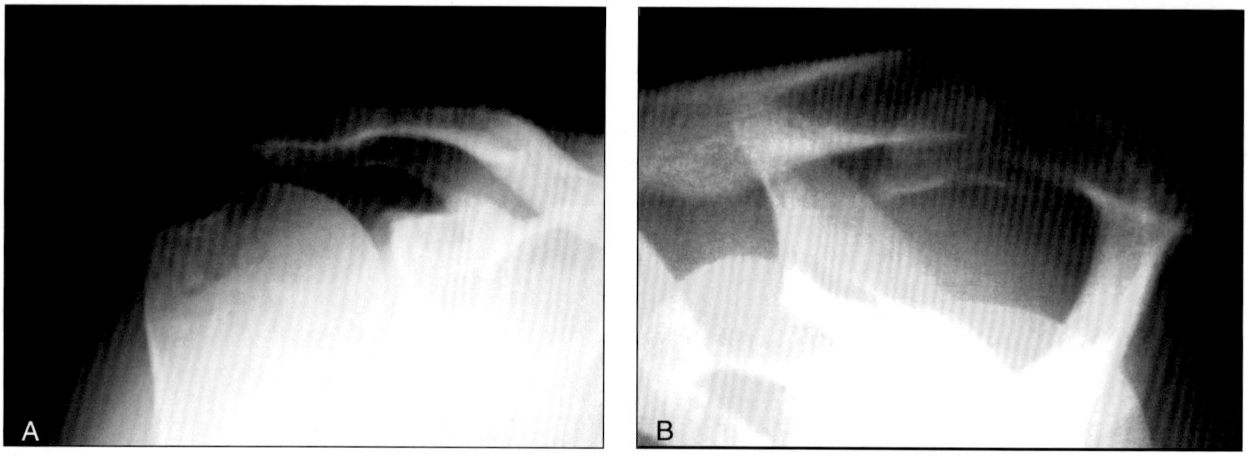

Figure 1 Preoperative AP **(A)** and outlet view **(B)** radiographs demonstrate subacromial and AC joint spur formation.

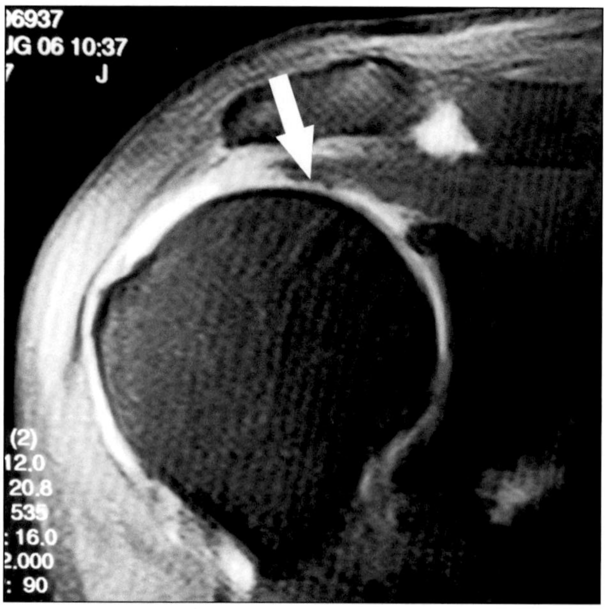

Figure 2 Coronal oblique MRI scan of the right shoulder reveals a medium-sized rotator cuff tear with retraction (arrow).

Arthroscopic acromioplasty, distal clavicle resection, rotator cuff repair, and biceps tenodesis were planned, and pump pressure was set at 60 mm Hg. The glenohumeral arthroscopy proceeded unremarkably with the débridement of the frayed biceps. Some bleeding was encountered upon entering the subacromial space, and the pump pressure was temporarily increased to approximately 100 mm Hg. The bleeding was controlled with a cautery device, and the pump pressure was reduced to 60 mm Hg. The surgeon then proceeded with the arthroscopic acromioplasty and distal clavicle resection (**Figure 5**), but additional bleeding occurred during the distal clavicle resection; thus, the pump pressure was temporarily increased to 100 mm Hg.

Mobilization of the rotator cuff began approximately 130 minutes into the procedure, and at this point the surgeon had more difficulty controlling bleeding. Despite the development of significant deltoid edema, the surgeon requested that the pump pressure be increased to 120 mm Hg. The patient, who had been conversing intermittently with the anesthesiologist, began to complain of some soreness in his throat and dysphagia. He reported that it "felt like a weight was on his neck," and he had greater difficulty breathing. The anesthesiologist examined the patient underneath the surgical drapes and noted significant swelling along the right side of the chest, the right side of the neck, and edema on the right side of the face. His skin was tense and cool, and he was becoming progressively diaphoretic and anxious. The blood pressure was now 200/120 mm Hg, and the anesthesiologist could not hear breath sounds clearly. The patient's oxygen saturation had dropped to 80%, despite the presence of the oxygen face shield, and continued to decrease to 75%. At this point, the anesthesiologist informed the surgeon that surgery must be temporarily stopped to control the patient's airway.

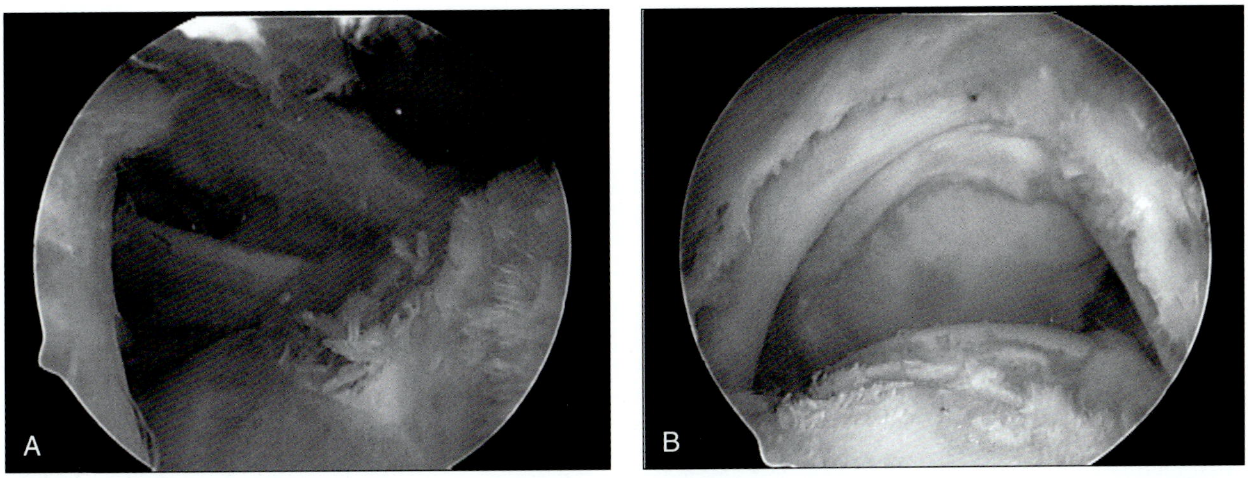

Figure 3 Arthroscopically, a large rotator cuff tear is visualized, with detachment of both the supraspinatus and infraspinatus tendons. The large tear is clearly visualized from the posterior portal **(A)** and from the mid-lateral portal **(B)**.

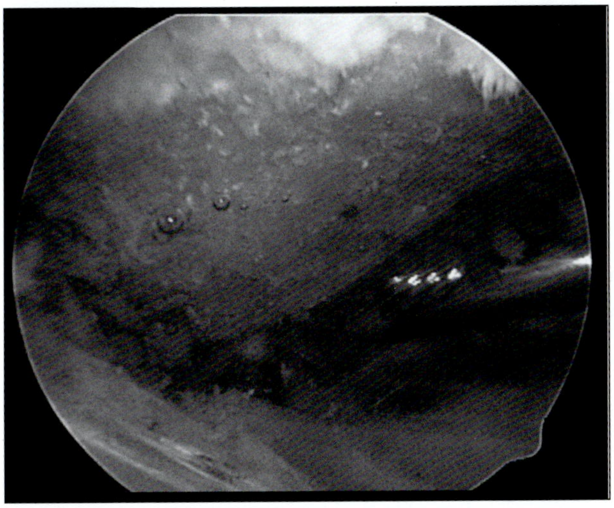

Figure 4 A large subacromial spur is visualized arthroscopically via the posterior portal.

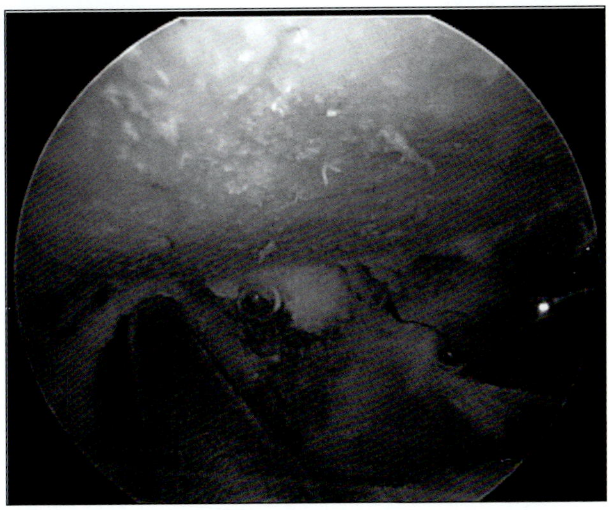

Figure 5 Arthroscopic visualization from the posterior portal reveals that the subacromial spur has been removed. The subacromial surface is now smooth.

Current Problem and Treatment

In this situation, a surgeon with average arthroscopic skills attempted to perform too many arthroscopic procedures at one time. Several factors led to the development of severe edema. Control of fluid extravasation during shoulder arthroscopy is critical to the success of the procedure but depends on many factors. In this case, severe fluid extravasation resulted in airway problems, necessitating emergent endotracheal intubation.

Discussion

Recognizing the Problem

Fluid overload following shoulder arthroscopy is relatively common, with severe problems noted in more than 2% of patients[1] (**Figure 6**). Lo and Burkhart[2] evaluated weight gain in patients following shoulder arthroscopy, noting an average increase of 8.7 ± 3.9

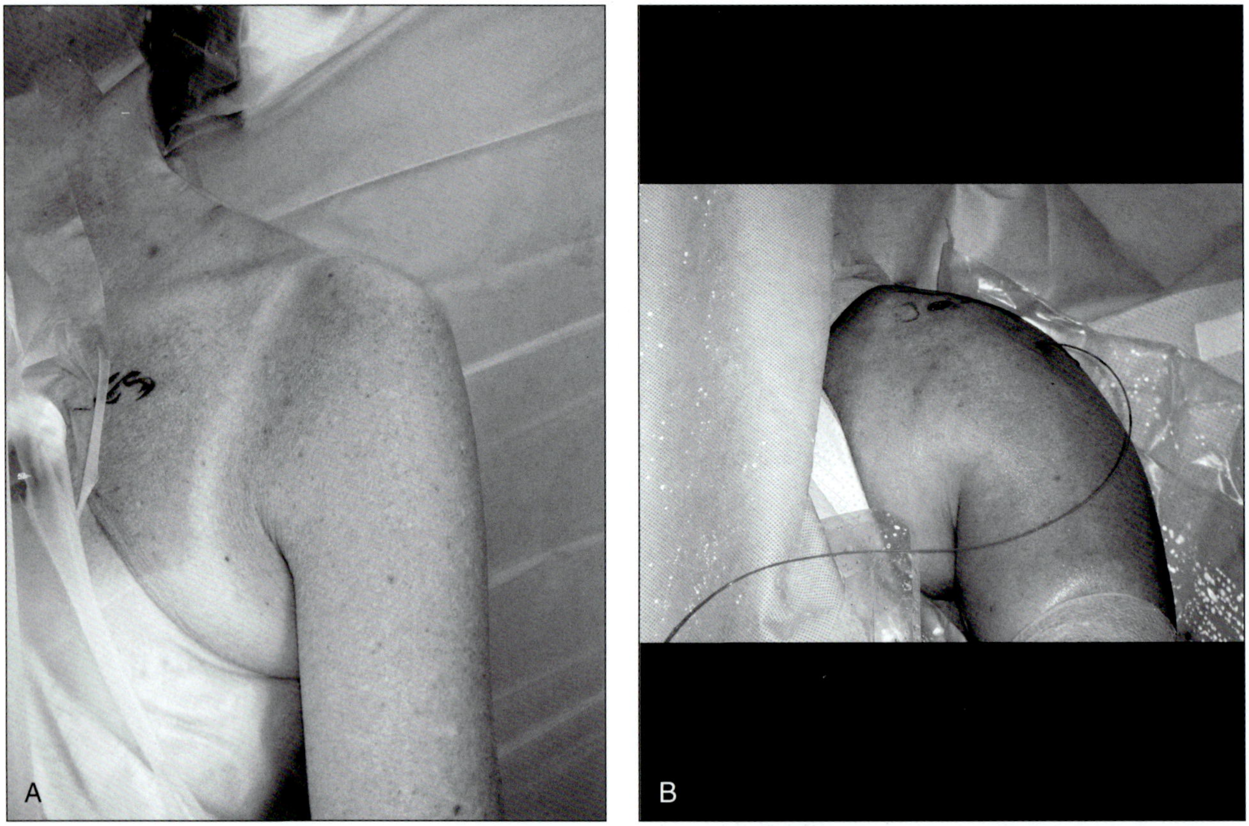

Figure 6 These clinical photos demonstrate typical edema, which can occur during the repair of a medium-sized rotator cuff tear performed in the beach chair position. Note the increase in size and loss of visual bony landmarks from preoperative **(A)** to postoperative **(B)**.

lb. More than 4 lb could be directly attributed to the infused arthroscopy fluid. In this series and others,[3] no complications were noted from this fluid absorption, and most commonly was an asymptomatic finding. Hynson and associates[4] reported that pulmonary edema developed in one of their patients following shoulder arthroscopy; postoperatively, their patient's urine output was 1,500 mL more than the total amount of intravenous fluid administered. The patient also had a 5-cm increase in neck circumference following shoulder arthroscopy performed in the beach chair position.

Causes of Fluid Overload

There are multiple causes for fluid overload during shoulder arthroscopy, but careful attention to detail can limit the volume of fluid administered and the severity of the fluid overload (**Table 1**).

The incidence of fluid overload is directly related to the duration of the procedure, with most series reporting a surgical time of more than 2 hours,[2,4,5] and to the complexity of the procedure and severity of the pathology. Fluid extravasation is more severe in patients with larger rotator cuff tears and in those with subscapularis involvement.[2]

The number of procedures attempted at the time of arthroscopy also is a factor. Surgical time is affected by surgeon proficiency: those who are experienced in arthroscopic surgery will be able to perform a procedure in less time than a surgeon who is not as experienced. The Arthroscopic Association of North America considers a surgeon who performs a minimum of 50 shoulder arthroscopies per year generally proficient in the technique.[6] Surgeons must be realistic about their proficiency to avoid this complication.

The amount of arthroscopic fluid needed to perform a procedure is another factor. Higher volumes of fluid result in increased edema, especially if the fluid is placed under high pressure by a pump and is leaking out of portals that are not secured with screw-in cannulas.[5,7] Pump pressures of less than 60 mm Hg are recommended for this reason.

Fluid extravasation is more severe when there is a loss of containment of closed spaces in the shoulder, particularly in patients with rotator cuff tears because fluid begins to extravasate out of the glenohumeral joint and into the subacromial and subdeltoid spaces immediately at the outset of surgery. This problem also can occur with capsular release when the glenohumeral joint capsule and rotator interval are released for scar contracture. Subacromial surgery is associated with fluid extravasation because the bursa does not provide a well-contained space,[8] especially when bursectomy is performed concomitantly with subacromial decompression. Inadvertent injury to the origin of the deltoid also has been associated with increased fluid extravasation because it provides another portal through which arthroscopic fluid can reach the subcutaneous tissue plane.[5]

Table 1 Risk Factors for Development of Edema During Shoulder Arthroscopy

1. Extended duration of procedure (longer than 2 hours)
2. High pump pressure
3. Loss of fluid containment (with subacromial surgery, rotator cuff repair, capsular release)
4. Obesity
5. Increased fluid volume

Patient Positioning Problems

Fluid extravasation most commonly leads to airway compression when the lateral decubitus position is used.[4] With the patient in this position, fluid tracks along tissue planes inferiorly toward the neck and chest wall and can lead to massive swelling of the neck, with tracheal deviation and airway obstruction. This complication also has been reported in the beach chair position in a case lasting more than 3 hours.[9] With the patient in an upright position, edema propagates inferiorly down the arm and onto the chest wall and is less likely to cause swelling in the neck. This problem is more severe in obese patients with a larger subcutaneous space.

Other Complications

Subcutaneous edema has been associated with other complications during shoulder arthroscopy. An increased incidence of neurologic deficit has been reported as a result of a combination of fluid edema and use of traction devices that can cause constriction around the arm.[10-12] Skin necrosis requiring skin grafting has been reported.[13] Although compartment syndrome of the leg has been associated with fluid extravasation from the knee,[14] there have been no reports of compartment syndrome in the shoulder. Pressure in the deltoid does rise during arthroscopy, but rapidly reverses upon removal of the inflow cannula, and relatively normal intracompartmental pressures of the deltoid are noted within 30 minutes of surgery.[3,15]

Airway Problems

Airway problems can develop for a variety of reasons during shoulder arthroscopy. Tension pneumothorax has been described intraoperatively[15] and may be related to puncture of the parietal pleura by either the arthroscope or a needle, or more commonly a ruptured alveolus caused by positive pressure ventilation. Pneumothorax also has been reported 1 day postoperatively in patients who are heavy smokers or have a history of asthma.[16] Pneumomediastinum and subcutaneous emphysema also have been reported[15,17] and may be related to extravasation of air up the axillary sheath to the thorax. This complication has been associated with the use of a positive pressure pump in combination with a suction shaver. Air is believed to be pulled into the joint by the shaver and then forced into the soft tissues by the pump mechanism. Negative pressure pulmonary edema also has been reported,[18] but has been clinically significant postoperatively rather than intraoperatively.

The differential diagnosis for airway problems during surgery includes hematoma from the interscalene block, phrenic nerve paralysis, anaphylaxis as a

Table 2 Tips for Avoiding Complications Caused by Severe Tissue Edema During Shoulder Arthroscopy

1. Limit the time of procedure to less than 2 hours; be prepared to convert to an open procedure if longer.
2. Surgical planning should take into consideration the surgeon's experience and skill, as well as the complexity of the patient's condition.
3. Consider use of airway adjuncts with the lateral decubitus position.
4. Minimize irrigation fluid pressure by using the following techniques:
   - hypotensive anesthesia
   - electrocautery for bleeding control
   - interscalene block
   - minimum pressure to provide visualization
   - avoid unrestricted drainage from portals

result of a drug reaction, high spinal block from administration of the interscalene block, and fluid extravasation. Reports of air embolism associated with gas distention in the joint include both lethal and nonlethal events resulting from cardiopulmonary collapse.[19-21]

Case Management Summary and Outcome

The arthroscopic instruments were removed and the wounds temporarily covered as the patient was placed in a supine position. Attempts at positive pressure ventilation with a face mask were unsuccessful, and the anesthesiologist determined that intubation was necessary. The patient was then sedated to allow intubation while awake. Laryngoscopy revealed massive swelling of the pharynx with only the tip of the epiglottis visible. A No. 6.0 endotracheal tube was passed blindly, and auscultation of breath sounds confirmed adequate positioning. Isofluorance was initiated, and the patient's oxygen saturation increased to 98%. The blood pressure was controlled, and a portable chest radiograph revealed soft-tissue swelling of the shoulder with tracheal deviation to the left. No pneumothorax was noted.

The patient was placed back into the lateral decubitus position, and the right arm was prepared again. At this point, the surgeon decided to finish the procedure through a mini-open approach. The edema had improved significantly within the 30 minutes it took to intubate the patient and reposition him. A deltoid splitting, mini-open approach was performed, and the rotator cuff was repaired using bone tunnels without complication. The biceps was tenodesed using a suture anchor.

Strategies to Minimize Common Complications

The development of severe edema and its related complications during surgery can be avoided with proper preparation (**Table 2**). All anatomic landmarks and portals should be marked on the skin preoperatively to avoid losing them should edema occur.

Careful monitoring of the arthroscopic fluid pressure is critical, and use of a pressure sensor on the arthroscope is valuable in preventing excessive pressure in the glenohumeral joint and subacromial space when a pump is used. Pressures should be monitored throughout the procedure and maintained at the lowest level possible while still maintaining visualization. Maneuvers such as use of hypotensive anesthesia, electrocautery to control bleeding, and cool arthroscopic fluids to encourage vasospasm allow pump pressure to be kept at a low level and are helpful in avoiding progressive edema.

Procedure time is limited in shoulder arthroscopy; therefore, the surgeon must be realistic about the complexity of the procedures attempted arthroscopically. Each surgeon should make a systematic transition from an all-open to an all-arthroscopic technique. Complications related to edema and fluid extravasation increase significantly in operations that last for more than 2 hours. An arthroscopic procedure should be aborted and converted to an open procedure if the operation cannot be performed within this time limit.

Screw-in cannulas can assist in preventing fluid extravasation out of the subacromial space and into the subcutaneous tissue plane. Use of these cannulas prevents uncontrolled flow of fluid from the portals, decreasing the amount of total irrigation fluid required to perform the arthroscopy.

Use of an interscalene block is beneficial because it allows shoulder arthroscopy to be performed without intubation. Intubation should be considered in complex procedures, with use of a lateral decubitus position, and if the patient is obese. Careful attention to airway patency is needed, given the potential that significant edema can occur around the neck and airway, particularly for surgeons who are less experienced in a particular procedure.

If the patient is not intubated for the procedure, both the surgeon and anesthesiologist must recognize the warning signs of pharyngeal edema. Loss of airway patency due to severe neck edema has been reported with use of a laryngeal mask airway, indicating that this device alone may not afford the needed protection against this complication.[22] In the event that an airway adjunct is not used, oversedation must be avoided because the patient will not be able to verbalize symptoms,[9] such as the sensation of a weight on the neck, any type of "sensation" in the throat, dysphagia, dyspnea, and difficulty speaking. Other observable signs that edema is reaching dangerous levels include swelling that extends into the face, neck, and chest.

Airway obstruction caused by fluid extravasation and pharyngeal edema can be a life-threatening problem; therefore, it is critical that the surgeon and anesthesiologist recognize the signs and symptoms.[9] If the patient is not intubated, both the anesthesiologist and surgeon should monitor the degree of swelling and the patient's airway status. In the event that airway compromise develops as a result of edema, emergency intubation may be necessary but extremely difficult secondary to swelling. The decision to complete the surgery depends on the stability of the patient's condition. In the intubated patient, the extent of the edema in the face, neck, and chest should be evaluated carefully prior to considering extubation. If significant pharyngeal edema is suspected, airway patency must be confirmed prior to extubation. Airway patency can be checked by releasing the cuff around the endotracheal tube, covering the lumen of the tube with a finger, and asking the patient to breathe.[4] Patients who cannot breathe independently should remain intubated until the edema resolves and should be monitored in a seated position to encourage dissipation of the edema fluid inferiorly. In most cases, pharyngeal swelling resolves within 12 hours, and the patient can be extubated.[5] Early extubation may be dangerous because edema around the neck may obscure normal anatomic landmarks and may make reintubation or even crycothyrotomy difficult.[23]

References

1. Berjano P, González BG, Olmedo JF, Perez-Espana LA, Munilla MG: Complications in arthroscopic shoulder surgery. *Arthroscopy* 1998;14:785-788.
2. Lo IK, Burkhart SS: Immediate postoperative fluid retention and weight gain after shoulder arthroscopy. *Arthroscopy* 2005;21:605-610.
3. Ogilvie-Harris DJ, Boynton E: Arthroscopic acromioplasty: Extravasation of fluid into the deltoid muscle. *Arthroscopy* 1990;6:52-54.
4. Hynson JM, Tung A, Guevara JE, Katz JA, Glick JM, Shapiro WA: Complete airway obstruction during arthroscopic shoulder surgery. *Anesth Analg* 1993;76:875-878.
5. Borgeat A, Bird P, Ekatodramis G, Dumont C: Tracheal compression caused by periarticular fluid accumulation: A rare complication of shoulder surgery. *J Shoulder Elbow Surg* 2000;9:443-445.
6. O'Neill PJ, Cosgarea AJ, Freedman JA, Queale WS, McFarland EG: Arthroscopic proficiency: A survey of orthopaedic sports medicine fellowship directors and orthopaedic surgery department chairs. *Arthroscopy* 2002;18:795-800.
7. Bigliani LU, Flatow EL, Deliz ED: Complications of shoulder arthroscopy. *Orthop Rev* 1991;20:743-751.
8. Matthews LS, Fadale PD: Subacromial anatomy for the arthroscopist. *Arthroscopy* 1989;5:36-40.
9. Orebaugh SL: Life-threatening airway edema resulting from prolonged shoulder arthroscopy. *Anesthesiology* 2003;99:1456-1458.
10. Rodeo SA, Forster RA, Weiland AJ: Neurological complications due to arthroscopy. *J Bone Joint Surg Am* 1993;75:917-926.
11. McFarland EG, O'Neill OR, Hsu CY: Complications of shoulder arthroscopy. *J South Orthop Assoc* 1997;6:190-196.
12. Standish WD, Peterson DC: Shoulder arthroscopy and nerve injury: Pitfalls and prevention. *Arthroscopy* 1995;11:458-466.
13. Mohammed KD, Hayes MG, Saies AD. Unusual complications of shoulder arthroscopy. *J Shoulder Elbow Surg* 2000;9:350-353.

14. Peek RD, Haynes DW: Compartment syndrome as a complication of arthroscopy. *Am J Sports Med* 1984;12:464-468.
15. Lee HC, Dewan N, Crosby L: Subcutaneous emphysema, pneumomediastinum, and potentially life-threatening tension pneumothorax: Pulmonary complications from arthroscopic shoulder decompression. *Chest* 1992;101:1265-1267.
16. Dietzel, DP, Ciullo JV: Spontaneous pneumothorax after shoulder arthroscopy: A report of four cases. *Arthroscopy* 1996;12:99-102.
17. Lau KY: Pneumomediastinum caused by subcutaneous emphysema in the shoulder: A rare complication of arthroscopy. *Chest* 1993;103:1606-1607.
18. Langan P, Michaels R: Negative-pressure pulmonary edema: A complication of shoulder arthroscopy. *Am J Orthop* 1999;28:56-58.
19. Faure EAM, Cook RI, Miles D: Air embolism during anesthesia for shoulder arthroscopy. *Anesthesiology* 1998;89:805-806.
20. Habegger R, Siebenmann R, Kieser C: Lethal air embolism during arthroscopy. *J Bone Joint Surg Br* 1989;71:314-316.
21. Hegde RT, Avatgere RN: Air embolism during anaesthesia for shoulder arthroscopy. *Br J Anaesth* 200;85:926-927.
22. Yoshimura E, Yano T, Ichinose K, Ushjjima K: Airway obstruction involving a laryngeal mask airway during arthroscopic shoulder surgery. *J Anesth* 2005;19:325-327.
23. Blumenthal S, Nadig M, Gerber C, Borgeat A: Severe airway obstruction during arthroscopic shoulder surgery. *Anesthesiology* 2003;99:1455-1456.

Chapter 3

Neurologic Deficit Following Shoulder Arthroscopy

Xavier A. Duralde, MD

Case Presentation

A 62-year-old right-handed male office worker is scheduled to undergo arthroscopic subacromial decompression and repair of a rotator cuff tear of the right shoulder that has failed to respond to nonsurgical treatment. Preoperative radiographs showed large spurs at the acromion and acromioclavicular (AC) joint (**Figure 1**), and MRI scans revealed a medium-sized, full-thickness rotator cuff tear (**Figure 2**).

Anesthesia plans included the combination of an interscalene block placed preoperatively and general anesthesia via an endotracheal tube. The interscalene block, consisting of 30 mL of 0.5% plain bupivacaine, was injected with the patient awake and after the anesthesiologist obtained a biceps twitch with the nerve stimulator set at a low setting. The patient was then intubated.

Initial Surgery

The surgery was performed with the patient in the beach chair position using a neurosurgical headrest. As the patient's skin was prepared for surgery, a belt was strapped around his waist to provide support on the operating table. The right arm was hung by a stockinette for preparation and draping and then placed in an arm holder for the procedure with gentle inferior and anterior traction applied.

Initial surgery consisted of arthroscopic acromioplasty, distal clavicle resection, and arthroscopic repair of the rotator cuff using suture anchors. Portals included a posterior "soft spot" portal, an anterior portal placed superior and lateral to the coracoid, and two lateral portals placed 2 cm and 3 cm inferior to the lateral acromion, respectively. The surgery proceeded without problems, and the patient was awakened and taken to the recovery room postoperatively in stable condition. The patient was then discharged home, reporting to be very comfortable with a dense block to the right arm.

The following day the patient presented to the office for a dressing change and wound check, reporting persistent dysesthesias along the radial aspect of the forearm radiating into the thumb. Sensation was restored to the rest of the arm. The patient described a "pins and needles" sensation affecting primarily the thumb and also reported moderate neck pain.

Physical examination revealed no signs of hematoma at the site of the interscalene block. Results of the Spurling test were mildly positive, with dysesthesias radiating down the arm along the C6 distribution. The Tinel sign at the wrist was negative, and the patient had a 2+ radial pulse with excellent capillary refill in the hand. There was no numbness in the upper arm and no skin changes in the forearm.

Shoulder radiographs showed adequate decompression of the subacromial space and AC joint, with the suture anchors clearly visualized in the greater tuberosity (**Figure 3**). Radiographs of the cervical spine showed multilevel spondylosis with disk space narrowing and osteophyte formation at C5-C6 and C6-C7 (**Figure 4**).

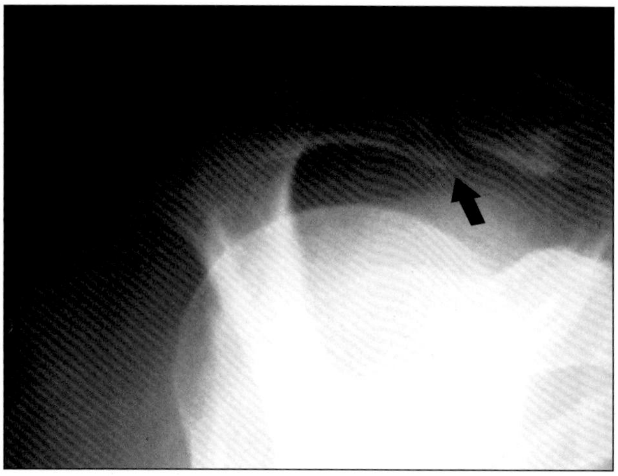

Figure 1 AP radiograph of the right shoulder reveals large spurs at the acromion and AC joint (arrow).

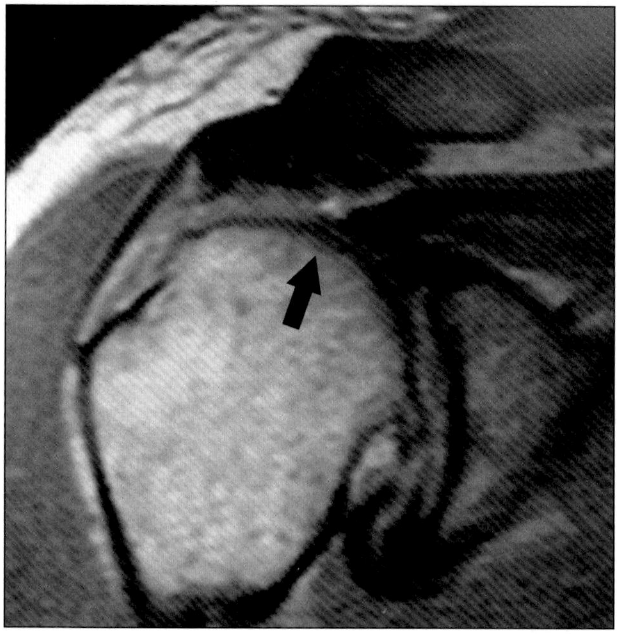

Figure 2 MRI scan reveals a medium-sized rotator cuff tear (arrow).

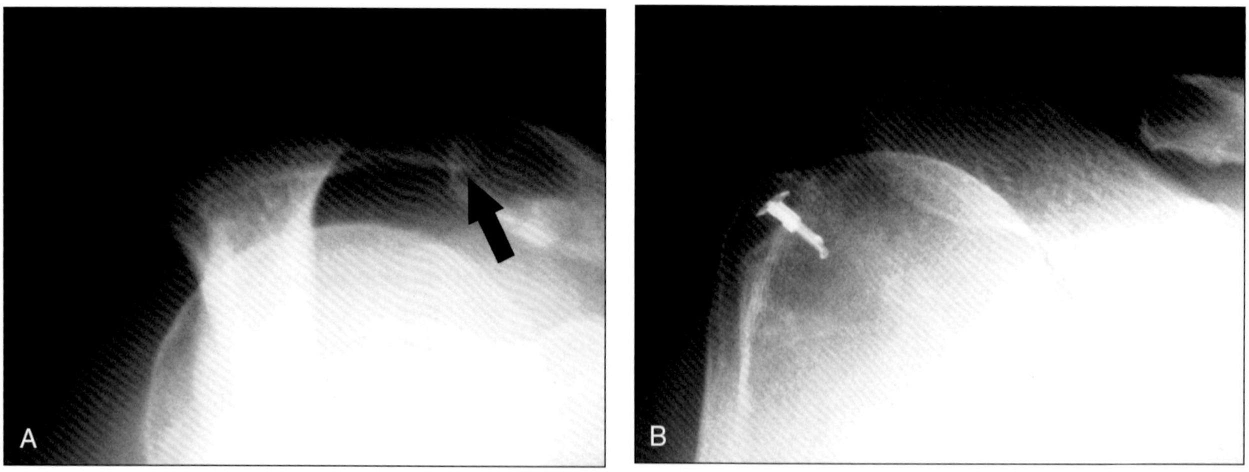

Figure 3 A and **B,** Postoperative radiographs demonstrate resection of the bone spurs. Note that the suture anchor is embedded in the greater tuberosity.

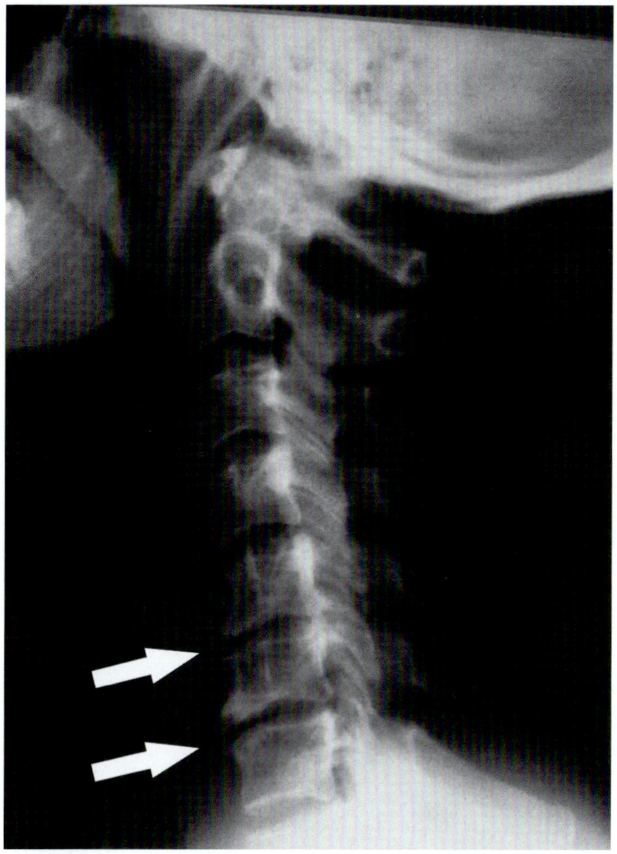

Figure 4 Lateral radiograph of the cervical spine reveals multilevel spondylosis at C5-C6 and C6-C7 (arrows).

Current Problem and Treatment

The patient has a neurologic deficit following otherwise unremarkable and successful shoulder arthroscopy. Nerve injuries following shoulder surgery represent one of the most worrisome problems for the surgeon because of the close proximity of the brachial plexus and multiple peripheral nerves to the operative field. The cervical spine also must be positioned properly to allow access to the shoulder without placing undue traction on the cervical nerve roots.

DISCUSSION

Recognizing Neurologic Injuries

Neurologic deficit following shoulder arthroscopy can be the result of a variety of factors. The nerve lesion could be in any number of locations, ranging from the cervical foramina to the carpal canal. Interventions associated with the procedure also can be a cause, which emphasizes the importance of meticulous attention to detail during every step of the procedure. The cause of the nerve injury in the case presentation may be associated with anesthetic techniques, events associated with positioning, or techniques associated with the surgery itself. Multiple precautionary steps, done both preoperatively and intraoperatively, can prevent these potentially disabling injuries. If a neurologic complication occurs, a thorough evaluation including physical examination, radiographs, and possibly electrophysiologic studies can help identify the location and the severity of the lesion and help direct treatment.

Table 1 Reported Neurologic Complications Associated With Shoulder Arthroscopy

1. Peripheral nerve injuries to the upper extremity
2. Femoral nerve injuries
3. Stroke
4. Carpal tunnel syndrome
5. Portal site injury
6. Brachial plexopathy
7. Seizures
8. Reflex sympathetic dystrophy
9. Quadriplegia

Neurologic injury associated with shoulder arthroscopy has been estimated to occur in up to 30% of patients.[1] A wide variety of neurologic complications has been reported in association with shoulder arthroscopy[1,2] (**Table 1**), and injuries to a surprisingly long list of nerves have been identified (**Table 2**). Most are neurapraxias that resolve within the first several months following surgery.[3] Hand or finger hypoesthesia or dysesthesia has a surprisingly extensive differential diagnosis both in terms of location of the nerve lesion as well as the cause (**Table 3**).

Patient Positioning

The beach chair and lateral decubitus positions for shoulder arthroscopy remain equally popular nationwide, and each is associated with specific nerve injuries.

Table 2 Reported Nerve Injuries Following Shoulder Arthroscopy

1. Central spinal cord lesions
2. Cervical radiculopathy
3. Brachial plexus lesions
4. Hypoglossal nerve injury
5. Axillary nerve injury
6. Musculocutaneous nerve injury
7. Lateral femoral cutaneous nerve injury
8. Ulnar nerve injury
9. Phrenic nerve injury
10. Radial nerve injury
11. Median nerve injury
12. Greater auricular nerve injury
13. Lesser occipital nerve injury
14. Medial pectoral nerve injury

Table 3 Differential Diagnosis for Hand Dysesthesias Following Shoulder Arthroscopy

1. Cervical radiculopathy secondary to neck positioning
2. Complications of the interscalene block
3. Residual interscalene block
4. Carpal tunnel syndrome due to suspension or traction device
5. Brachial plexus stretch due to traction
6. Tourniquet effect resulting from the position of the arm holder or traction device
7. Nerve injury at a portal

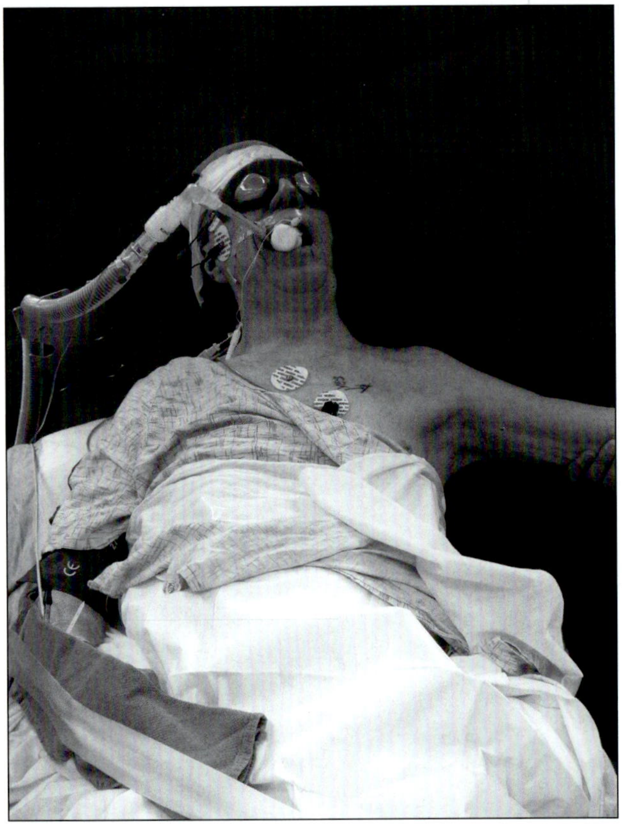

Figure 5 Traction on the operative arm in a patient in the beach chair position can cause injury to the brachial plexus if the trunk is allowed to shift on the table with the head fixed.

Nerve injuries associated with the beach chair position include hypoglossal nerve injury,[4] lesser occipital nerve injury,[5] and cervical radiculopathy (personal experience). Brachial plexus injuries seem to be associated with neck extension, rotation, and lateral flexion, which can occur when arm traction is applied during the procedure and the patient's head is fixed on the headrest but the trunk shifts toward the surgeon (**Figure 5**). This position is most likely to occur with instability repair in which distraction of the humeral head away from the glenoid is critical for visualization of the capsule and labrum anteroinferiorly.[6] Cervical root lesions are more likely to occur if the patient's trunk shifts away from the operative shoulder, leading to lateral flexion of the neck and foraminal narrowing on the operative side[6] (**Figure 6**). In these cases, some type of bolster or wrap should be considered to limit movement of the patient's trunk on the table if traction is necessary (**Figure 7**).

Patients at the greatest risk for cervical radiculopathy are those with preexisting cervical spondylosis, as described in the case presentation. A neurosurgical headrest is useful in facilitating neutral positioning of the neck and stabilization of the head on the table while allowing full access to the shoulder. Fixing the patient's head to a lower profile bolster or to the operating table itself with the patient in the beach chair position does not adequately compensate for thoracic lordosis and results in cervical extension with further closure of cervical foramina.

Also with the beach chair position, the median nerve is at risk for injury if the arm is hung from a stockinette preoperatively during preparation. A tight band should not be placed along the volar aspect of the wrist during this maneuver (**Figure 8**).

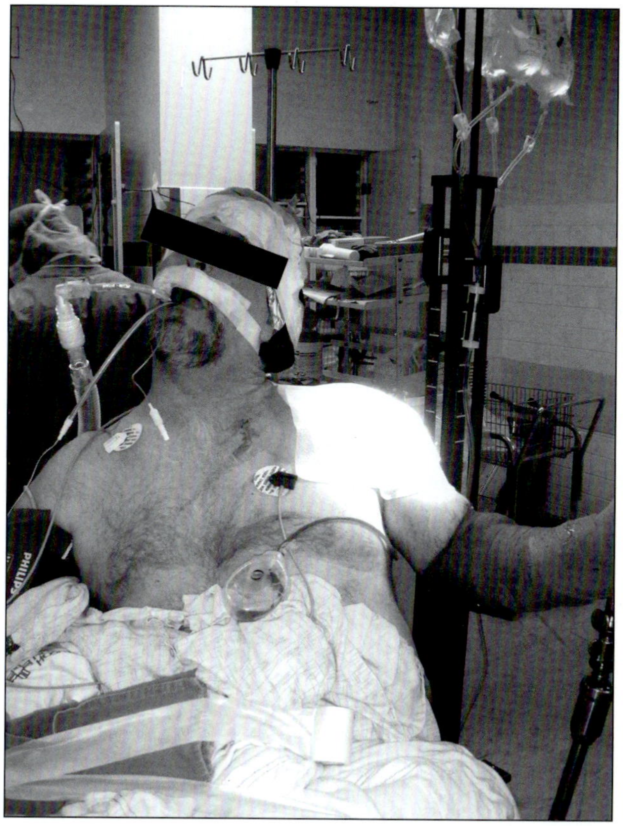

Figure 6 If the patient's body shifts away from the operative side, lateral flexion of the neck may lead to increased pressure on the nerve roots on the operative side.

The hand can be hung from a loop, placing pressure on the dorsum of the wrist but avoiding any pressure to the carpal canal. Careful attention to proper patient positioning can reduce the risk of complications in the beach chair position (**Table 4; Figure 9**).

The lateral decubitus position is much more commonly associated with nerve injury than the beach chair position,[7] and great care is needed in positioning the patient on the table and in positioning the traction device on the operative arm (**Table 5; Figure 10**). Use of an axillary roll is critical for protecting the nerves of the dependent, nonoperative arm during the procedure. The patient's head should be in neutral position, avoiding lateral flexion toward the operating table, which will increase traction on the brachial plexus of the operative arm. Several authors have evaluated the strain on the brachial plexus in the lateral decubitus position during shoulder arthroscopy.[8,9]

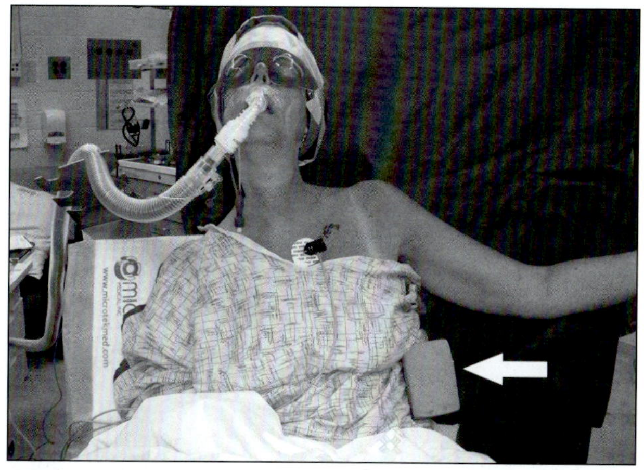

Figure 7 With the beach chair position, a chest bolster (arrow) or sheet wrapped around the table will limit trunk motion and protect the brachial plexus during arthroscopic surgery.

Table 4 Tips for Avoiding Complications With the Beach Chair Position

1. Place the neck in a neutral position in the neurosurgical headrest.
2. Avoid tight straps across the iliac crest.
3. Use caution when hanging arm for preparation or placement in a traction device to avoid pressure on the carpal canal.
4. Avoid displacement of the trunk by excessive traction on arm.
5. Pad and secure the contralateral arm.
6. Pad the heels and place a pillow underneath the knees.
7. Avoid excess edema.

Table 5 Tips for Avoiding Complications in the Lateral Decubitus Position

1. Pad dependent side using an axillary roll.
2. Pad the fibular head and lateral malleolus.
3. Avoid too much pressure to the iliac crest.
4. Avoid extension of operative arm in traction; the ideal position is 20° of flexion and less than 70° of abduction.
5. Avoid excessive traction; limit longitudinal traction to 10 lb to 20 lb and vertical traction to less than 7 lb.
6. Avoid excessive edema.
7. Secure the trunk in a lateral position; forward trunk roll will result in arm extension.
8. Maintain the neck in a neutral position; avoid lateral flexion toward the operating table.

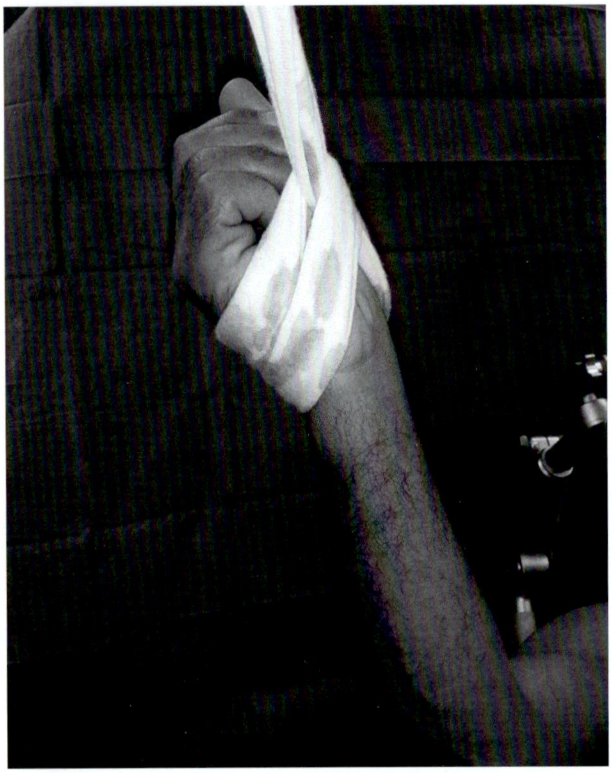

Figure 8 If the arm is hung from a stockinette for preparation, pressure at the carpal canal must be avoided.

The musculocutaneous nerve is at greatest risk when the patient is in the lateral decubitus position during shoulder arthroscopy, and neurapraxias are associated with arm position, degree of fluid extravasation during surgery, and amount of traction applied to the arm during surgery. Tension is greatest on the brachial plexus with extension and adduction of the arm. Arm positions between 20° and 45° of flexion and less than 70° of abduction generally are recommended to minimize nerve injury in this position.[6,8-10] Extension must be avoided. Arm traction should be limited to 10 lb to 20 lb of longitudinal traction and no more than 7 lb of vertical traction. Abduction of the arm lateralizes the positions of the axillary and musculocutaneous nerves, making them more vulnerable to injury at portal sites.

Arm wraps used with traction devices in either the beach chair or lateral decubitus position can lead to a tourniquet effect, especially in cases associated with extravasation of fluid, and may lead to direct nerve compression. Potential for nerve injury represents one of the many reasons to avoid severe edema during surgery.

Portal Creation

Standard arthroscopic portals generally are safe with regard to proximity to peripheral nerves.[11] Although it is safe to create these portals using an outside-in technique, the surgeon must be aware of surface anatomy and the relative location and pathways of the nerves in the region.[12] Anterior portals should be kept superior and lateral to the coracoid to avoid injury to the brachial plexus, axillary nerve, and musculocutaneous nerve (**Figure 11**, *A*). Anterior, anterosuperior, and even anteroinferior portals[13] passing through the subscapularis are all a safe distance away from these structures. Increased abduction and edema from fluid extravasation can alter the locations of these nerves, placing them at risk for injury. Matthews and associates[14] described a proximal median nerve injury from direct injury at the anterior portal. The posterior portal is 2 cm away from both the suprascapular nerve and the axillary nerve (**Figure 11**, *B*). Inferior angulation of a trocar from the posterior portal can result in damage to the axillary nerve and the posterior humeral circumflex vessels. A medially directed trocar from the posterior portal can similarly damage the suprascapular nerve. The lateral portal has been associated with damage to sensory branches of the axillary nerve with variable patterns of dysesthesia along the lateral and medial upper arm.[3]

Anesthesia Issues

An interscalene block is generally considered a safe, effective means of anesthesia and preemptive analgesia.[15] The success rate of the interscalene block varies between 92% and 98% in the hands of experienced anesthesiologists[16,17] and is associated with a very high level of patient satisfaction because of its exceptional analgesic effects in the perioperative period. Neurapraxias have been associated with this form of anesthesia in up to 4.5% of patients,[16,18] but most resolve within the first several months following surgery. The incidence of neurapraxia from

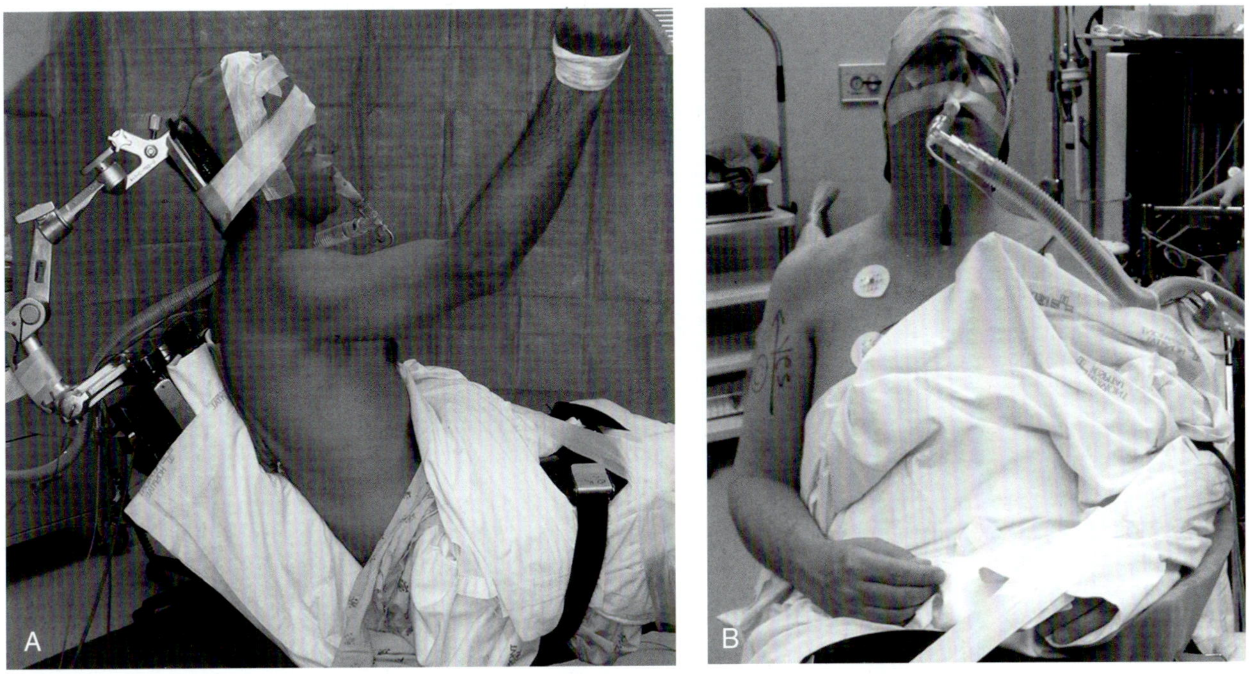

Figure 9 A, Proper beach chair positioning as viewed from the side. Careful attention to detail is required to avoid complications when positioning the patient in the beach chair position. Follow the tips in Table 4 to avoid placing excessive stress on the nerves in the cervical spine, operative arm, nonoperative arm, and lower extremities. Note the neck position and head control as well as the use of safety straps and an arm holder. **B,** Proper beach chair positioning as viewed from the front. Note that the nonoperative arm is well-padded and secured. A safety strap is placed across the thighs; the tightness of the strap is rechecked after sitting the patient upright to avoid placing excessive pressure on the lateral femoral cutaneous nerves.

an interscalene block can be minimized by use of a nerve stimulator to obtain paresthesias prior to injection and applying the block in an awake patient to minimize the possibility of an intraneural injection. Other neurologic sequelae of the interscalene block include high spinal anesthesia and generalized seizures, both of which are serious (and extremely rare) but can be handled safely in a monitored operating room setting. Preoperative placement of the block reduces the required amount of anesthetic needed during the procedure and has many other benefits, including decreased bleeding, reduced time to discharge from the postanesthesia care unit, and excellent postoperative analgesia.[19]

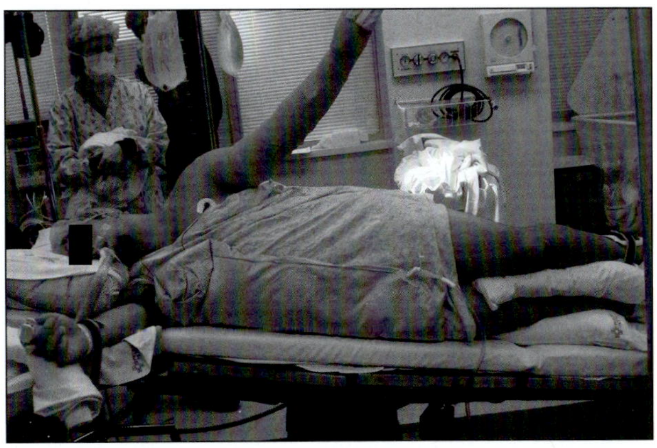

Figure 10 Body padding and positioning, as well as arm traction position and weight, are critical in avoiding complications in the lateral decubitus position. See Table 5 for details.

Associated Surgical Interventions

The incidence of neurologic injuries following shoulder arthroscopy also is directly proportional

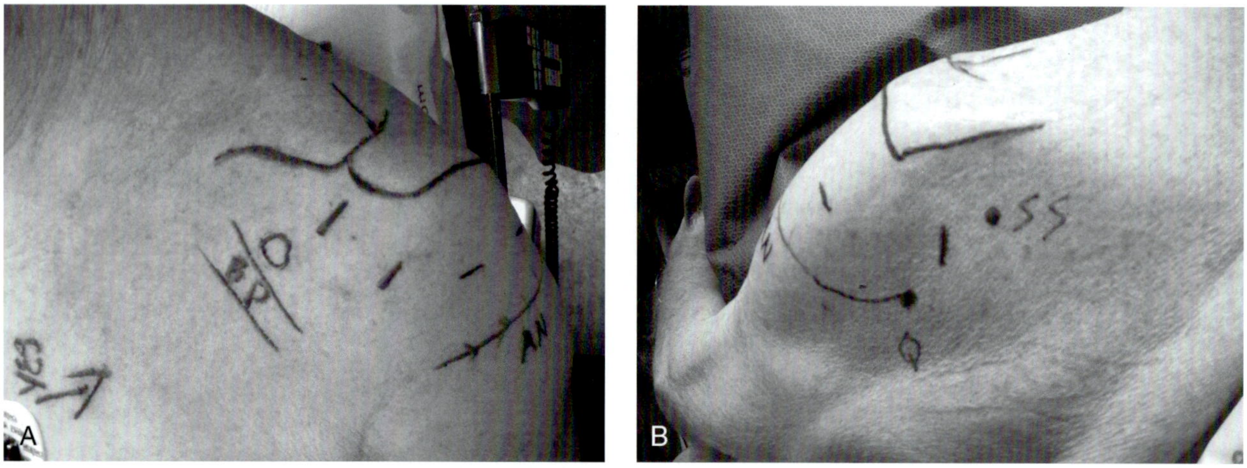

Figure 11 Standard arthroscopic portals are generally kept a safe distance from neuromuscular structures, but the location of these structures must be kept in mind throughout the procedure. **A,** Anterior view. The two anterior portals, shown as straight lines, are placed superior and lateral to the coracoid (marked as a circle). They are a safe distance from the positions of the brachial plexus (BP) and the axillary nerve (AN), which have been marked. **B,** Posterior view. The posterior and lateral portals are shown as straight lines. Note the distance away from the suprascapular nerve (SS) and the quadrilateral space (Q), which is the exit point for the axillary nerve. The axillary nerve passes from posterior to anterior on the undersurface of the deltoid, approximately 5 cm distal to the lateral edge of the acromion. This is a safe distance from the lateral portals.

to the complexity of the surgery, and this complication occurs more often with certain procedures.[7] Thermal capsulorrhaphy has fallen out of favor over the past several years because of variable results and significant complications.[20] Axillary neurapraxia has been commonly reported with this procedure as a result of direct thermal trauma to the nerve as it passes inferior to the joint in intimate contact with the capsule.

Arthroscopic capsular release requires release of the inferior capsule in close proximity to the axillary nerve, but, surprisingly, there have been no reports of axillary nerve damage associated with this surgery.[21] Excessively medial dissection and release of a retracted rotator cuff can damage the suprascapular nerve, and release at the level of the scapular spine must be performed with extreme caution. Simple subacromial decompressions have been associated with a much lower rate of neurologic injuries.[22]

Other Neurologic Lesions

Neurologic lesions have been reported in other areas of the body during shoulder arthroscopy and are generally related to positioning. In the lateral decubitus position, the fibular head and lateral malleolus must be padded to avoid injury to the peroneal nerve. An axillary roll is critical for avoiding neurologic problems in the contralateral arm. Meralgia paresthetica can occur if the safety belt is too tight across the iliac crests on patients in the beach chair position. This complication occurs if the belt is applied before the patient is moved from the supine to the beach chair position. If the belt is not loosened, and pressure is placed across the iliac crest during surgery, the patient may awaken with dysesthesias of the lateral femoral cutaneous nerve. This complication also has been reported with the lateral decubitus position from direct pressure between the iliac crest and the operating table.

Case Management and Outcome Summary

The working diagnosis for this patient was cervical radiculopathy associated with neck positioning at the time of surgery. The patient was given a prescription for pregabalin and advised to observe symptoms over the next week. The patient called back 1 week later, reporting that the symptoms had become more severe and the dysesthesias were worse at night and only partially responsive to medication.

MRI scans obtained at this time revealed a C5-C6 disk osteophyte complex with moderate compression of the right C6 nerve root (**Figure 12**). Physical examination at this time was unchanged, with patient reports of dysesthesias but no detectable motor deficit. Based on the physical examination findings and MRI scans, a selective nerve root injection of corticosteroids was ordered, with complete resolution of symptoms. The postoperative course was otherwise unremarkable.

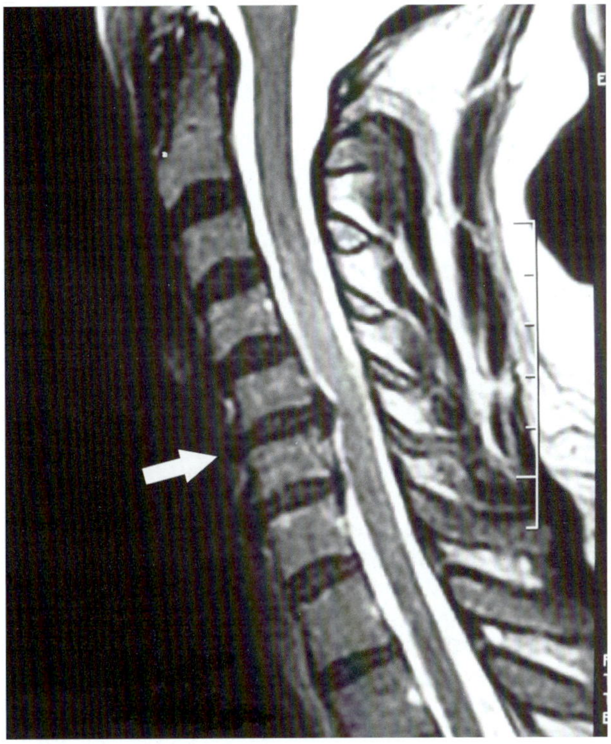

Figure 12 MRI scan of the cervical spine reveals a C5-C6 disk osteophyte complex with moderate compression of the right C6 nerve root, which correlates with the patient's symptom complex.

Strategies to Minimize Common Complications

Most neurologic deficits following shoulder arthroscopy are temporary neurapraxias that resolve with observation.[3] Nevertheless, thorough physical and radiographic examinations are indicated to identify the site of the nerve lesion and assist with treatment. A positive Spurling test and distributions of paresthesias along a dermatomal distribution suggest a radicular problem.

Characteristic patterns of sensory loss can help guide the surgeon in instances of peripheral nerve injury. The axillary nerve is associated with sensory loss both in the medial and lateral aspects of the upper arm.[3] The sensory branch of the musculocutaneous nerve is the lateral antebrachial cutaneous nerve with a sensory distribution along the lateral forearm. The sensory distribution of the median nerve is along the volar aspect of the hand radially. Specific muscle groups can be evaluated for weakness, although this examination may be limited in the perioperative period because of pain.

Radiographic evaluation should include cervical spine radiographs to rule out spondylosis, and in patients with radicular findings on physical examination, MRI of the cervical spine should be performed. Electrophysiologic changes, which can be detected on electromyographic/nerve conduction velocity studies, typically do not develop until approximately 4 to 6 weeks following nerve injury. Therefore, these studies should not be ordered unless significant neurologic deficit is noted beyond the 6-week mark.

The most common treatment for a neurologic injury following shoulder arthroscopy is observation and adherence to the planned postoperative protocol for the shoulder surgery performed. Medications such as gabapentin and pregabalin may improve comfort for patients with paresthesias. If a radicular source of the nerve injury is suspected and the patient has had persistent paresthesias for more than 2 weeks postoperatively, MRI is beneficial for ruling out nerve root compression. Cervical epidural steroid injection or selective nerve root injections of corticosteroids also may be beneficial in this instance. Surgical decompression has not been required for radicular symptoms following shoulder arthroscopy. Reexploration of the shoulder is indicated only in instances in which entrapment of a nerve by suture is suspected.

References

1. McFarland EG, O'Neill OR, Hsu CY: Complications of shoulder arthroscopy. *J South Orthop Assoc* 1997;6:190-196.
2. Segmüller HE, Alfred SP, Zilio G, Saies AD, Hayes MG: Cutaneous nerve lesions of the shoulder and arm after arthroscopic shoulder surgery. *J Shoulder Elbow Surg* 1995;4:254-258.
3. Rodeo SA, Forster RA, Weiland AJ: Neurologic complications due to arthroscopy. *J Bone Joint Surg Am* 1993;75:917-926.
4. Mullins RC, Drez D Jr, Cooper J: Hypoglossal nerve palsy after arthroscopy of the shoulder and open operation with the patient in the beach chair position: A case report. *J Bone Joint Surg Am* 1992;74:137-139.
5. Park TS, Kim YS: Neuropraxia of the cutaneous nerve of the cervical plexus after shoulder arthroscopy. *Arthroscopy* 2005;21:631.
6. Stanish WD, Peterson DC: Shoulder arthroscopy and nerve injury: Pitfalls and prevention. *Arthroscopy* 1995;11:458-466.
7. Bigliani LU, Flatow EL, Deliz ED: Complications of shoulder arthroscopy. *Orthop Rev* 1991;20:743-751.
8. Klein AH, France JC, Mutschler TA, Fu FH: Measurement of brachial plexus strain in arthroscopy of the shoulder. *Arthroscopy* 1987;3:45-52.
9. Pitman MI, Nainzedeh N, Ergas E, Springer S: The use of somatosensory evoked potentials for detection of neuropraxia during shoulder arthroscopy. *Arthroscopy* 1988;4:250-255.
10. Andrews JR, Carson WG Jr, Ortega K: Arthroscopy of the shoulder: Technique and normal anatomy. *Am J Sports Med* 1984;12:1-7.
11. Lo IK, Lind CC, Burkhart SS: Glenohumeral arthroscopy portals established using an outside-in technique: Neurovascular anatomy at risk. *Arthroscopy* 2004;20:596-602.
12. Nottage WM: Arthroscopic portals: Anatomy at risk. *Orthop Clin N Am* 1993;24:19-26.
13. Davidson PA, Tibone JE: Anterior-inferior (5 o'clock) portal for shoulder arthroscopy. *Arthroscopy* 1995;11:519-525.
14. Matthews LS, Zarins B, Michael RH, Helfet DL: Anterior portal selection for shoulder arthroscopy. *Arthroscopy* 1985;1:33-39.
15. Brown AR, Weiss R, Greenberg C, Flatow EL, Bigliani LU: Interscalene block for shoulder arthroscopy: Comparison with general anesthesia. *Arthroscopy* 1993;9:295-300.
16. Bishop JY, Sprague M, Gelber J, Krol M, Rosenblatt MA, Gladstone JN, Flatow EL: Interscalene regional anesthesia for arthroscopic shoulder surgery: A safe and effective technique. *J Shoulder Elbow Surg* 2006;15:567-570.
17. Faryniarz D, Morelli C, Coleman S, Holmes T, Allen A, Altchek D, Cordasco F, Warren RF, Urban MK, Gordon MA: Interscalene block anesthesia at an ambulatory surgery center performing predominantly regional anesthesia: A prospective study of one hundred thirty-three patients undergoing shoulder surgery. *J Shoulder Elbow Surg* 2006;15:686-690.
18. Candido KD, Sukhani R, Doty R Jr, Nader A, Kendall MC, Yaghmour E, Kataria TC, McCarthy R: Neurologic sequelae after interscalene brachial plexus block for shoulder/upper arm surgery: The association of patient, anesthetic, and surgical factors to the incidence and clinical course. *Anesth Analg* 2005;100:1489-1495.
19. Hadzic A, Williams BA, Karaca PE, Hobeika P, Unis G, Dermksian J, Yufa M, Thys DM, Santos AC: For outpatient rotator cuff surgery, nerve block anesthesia provides superior same-day recovery over general anesthesia. *Anesthesiology* 2005;102:1001-1007.
20. Wong KL, Williams GR: Complications of thermal capsulorrhaphy of the shoulder. *J Bone Joint Surg Am* 2001;83(suppl 2 pt 2):151-155.
21. Price MR, Tillett ED, Acland RD, Nettleton GS: Determining the relationship of the axillary nerve to the shoulder joint capsule from an arthroscopic perspective. *J Bone Joint Surg Am* 2004;86:2135-2142.
22. Paulos LE, Franklin JL: Arthroscopic shoulder decompression development and application: A five year experience. *Am J Sports Med* 1990;18:235-244.

Chapter 4

Failure of Arthroscopic Rotator Cuff Repair

Donald P. Endrizzi, MD

Case Presentation

Case 1

A 52-year-old female teacher presented with a 9-month history of pain over the lateral aspect of her right shoulder. The pain was particularly troublesome at night, often disturbing her sleep, and she noted difficulty writing on the chalkboard. The onset was insidious but was initially attributed to her weight-training exercise program. Trials of nonsteroidal anti-inflammatory drugs and physical therapy provided no relief. Her primary care physician recommended a corticosteroid injection, which improved her symptoms for approximately 4 weeks.

On physical examination, the patient's shoulders appeared symmetric and without atrophy. Her cervical spine moved freely, with no discomfort. Active and passive range of motion revealed forward flexion to 170°, external rotation to 60°, and internal rotation to T9. She had good strength of internal and external rotation. Lift-off and abdominal-compression tests for subscapularis deficiency were negative, but Neer and Hawkins impingement signs were markedly positive.

Radiographs revealed no glenohumeral arthrosis, but the supraspinatus outlet view showed a type 2 acromion (**Figure 1**). An MRI scan showed a full-thickness rotator cuff tear limited to the supraspinatus muscle, with minimal retraction.

Initial Surgery

The patient underwent arthroscopic rotator cuff repair, with an acromioplasty. The tear was repaired using two Mason-Allen stitches and bioabsorbable suture anchors. Postoperative radiographs revealed an adequate acromioplasty, with no other abnormalities (**Figure 2**). She was immobilized in a sling for 6 weeks and began a limited passive range-of-motion program supervised by a physical therapist at 2 weeks postoperatively. Active motion was started at 6 weeks and gentle strengthening exercises at 10 weeks.

Current Problem and Treatment

By 12 weeks postoperatively, the patient recovered nearly all of her preoperative motion; however, she still had daily pain that was similar in character to her preoperative pain. She remarked that the pain continued to disturb her sleep and interfere with activities of daily living.

Physical examination revealed well-healed arthroscopy portals, with slight atrophy of the supraspinatus. Active and passive range of motion was similar to the preoperative findings. Impingement signs were positive, and pain was elicited with strength testing. Laboratory studies, including a complete blood cell count, C-reactive protein level, and erythrocyte sedimentation rate, were within normal limits. MRI scans showed failure of the rotator cuff repair, with loss of fixation at the suture-tendon interface (**Figure 3**). The patient elected to proceed with arthroscopic revision surgery.

DISCUSSION

Recognizing the Problem

Although numerous studies have demonstrated high rates of success, arthroscopic rotator cuff repair is not always successful. Complications of arthroscopic rotator cuff repair are similar to those of open rotator cuff repair and include stiffness, failure to heal, infection, reflex sympathetic dystrophy, deep

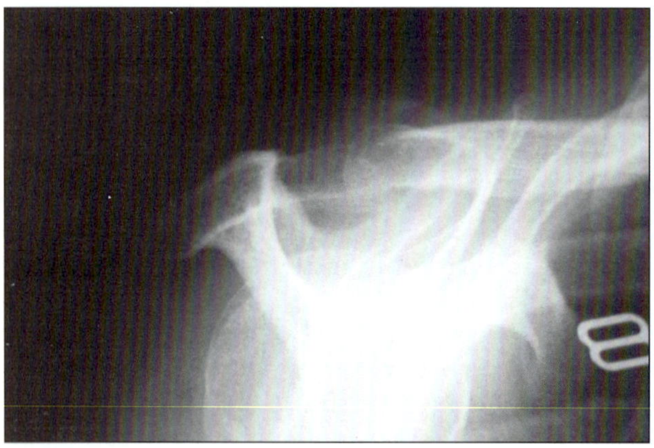

Figure 1 Preoperative outlet view shows a type II acromion.

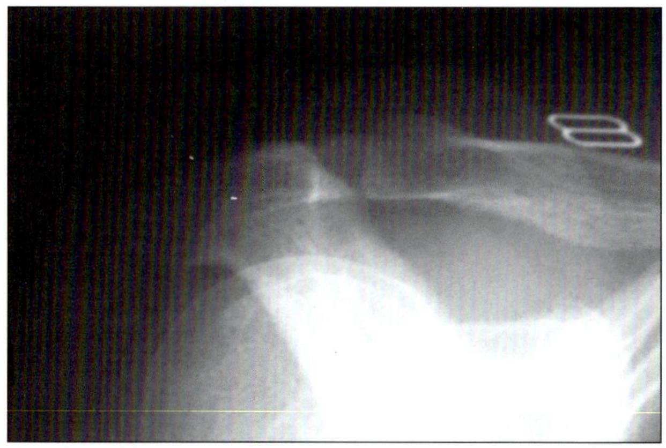

Figure 2 Postoperative outlet view.

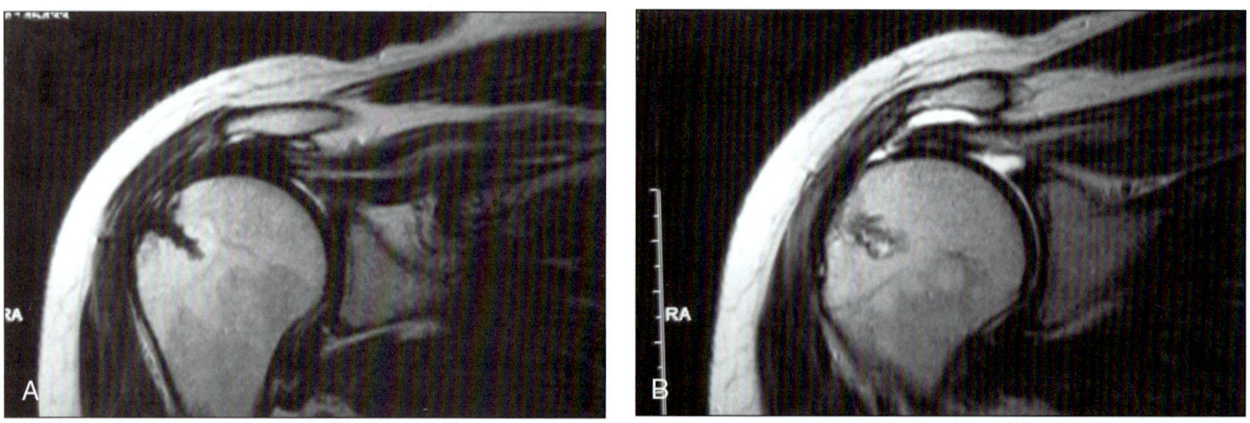

Figure 3 Postoperative MRI scans showing the suture anchor remaining in bone but failure of the repair.

vein thrombosis, and even death[1] (**Table 1**). Fortunately, many of these complications are exceedingly rare, but failure to heal remains problematic.

The patient's 12-week postoperative radiographs revealed subtle evidence of erosion at the greater tuberosity and acromion that were not present on the initial postoperative radiographs (**Figure 4**). These findings suggest some inflammatory or mechanical process at the site of the repair. Postoperative infection, inflammatory response to the anchor or suture material, and mechanical erosion subsequent to anchor pullout are possible causes.

Postoperative Infection

Any evaluation for failed rotator cuff surgery must consider postoperative infection as a cause. Infection can lead to suture anchor loosening and eventual failure of the repair. Most postoperative infections develop within 3 to 6 weeks after rotator

Table 1: Complications of Rotator Cuff Repair

Misdiagnosis
- Cervical spine disease
- Neuropathies
- AC pathology
- Biceps pathology
- Instability and labral pathology
- Glenohumeral arthritis
- Adhesive capsulitis

Surgical Failure
- Stiffness
- Rerupture or failure to heal
- Loss of fixation
- Infection
- Nerve Injury
- Complex regional pain syndrome
- Deep vein thrombosis

General Arthroscopic Complications
- Transient traction neurapraxia
- Extravasation
- Anesthesia-related complications

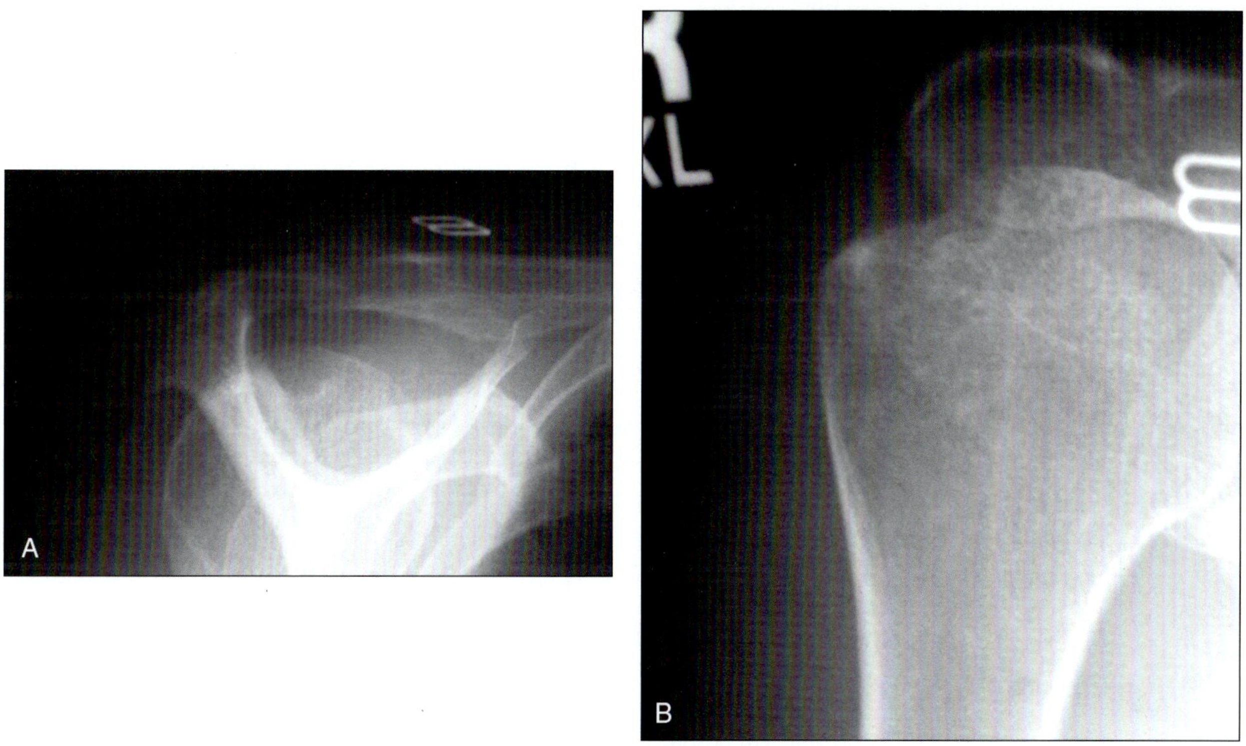

Figure 4 Radiographs at 12 weeks reveal some erosion at the greater tuberosity and acromion that were not present on the initial postoperative radiographs.

cuff surgery, with *Propionibacterium acnes*, a normal skin bacterium, as a frequent causative organism.[2] Infections caused by low-virulence organisms such as *P acnes* may be more indolent. Laboratory studies will usually show an elevated C-reactive protein level and erythrocyte sedimentation rate; however, the complete blood cell count may be within normal limits.

Suture Anchor Pullout

Inflammatory responses to suture anchor materials have been rarely reported,[3] but may cause cyst formation and bone resorption, resulting in suture anchor loosening and pullout. However, when it occurs, failure at the anchor-bone interface is more likely associated with poor bone quality or poor initial bone fixation.

When anchor pullout occurs, it may be difficult to differentiate symptoms of a normal postoperative course versus failure of cuff fixation. Bioabsorbable anchors are radiolucent, making it impossible to locate them on plain radiographs when fixation fails; however, the presence of erosions on plain films suggests the possibility of anchor displacement. Metallic anchors, by contrast, are easily seen on plain radiographs but can obscure visualization of the repair if a subsequent MRI scan is needed.

Preventing Fixation Failures

Strength of Suture Anchor Fixation

The strength of suture anchor fixation at the greater tuberosity depends on many factors, including bone mineral density,[4] presence of bone cysts,[5] and prior anchor placement. These factors must be considered when selecting the location or type of suture anchor to use in the fixation.

The surgeon should choose the fixation device carefully. Different suture anchor designs vary in holding power—for example, because of differences in thread depth and pitch in screw-type anchors or expansion in friction-fit designs.[4,6,7] Additionally, some authors suggest that the anchor insertion angle, or "deadman's angle," may improve anchor pullout strength, but there is some debate as to its importance.[8] There is no agreement in the literature on which size of suture anchor to use for rotator cuff fixation, but most authors suggest a 4.0-mm or larger anchor. Anchors should be spaced 1.0 cm to 1.5 cm apart to allow for adequate bone bridging between anchors. Spacing the anchors too far apart may not provide secure fixation or recreate an adequate cuff footprint for healing. No consensus exists regarding knot tying, knot types, or knotless designs.

Configuration of Suture Anchor Placement

The number of anchors used may also increase the strength of fixation. Several recent studies have addressed the importance of increasing the footprint of the repaired tendon to the bone using various configurations of anchor and suture placement. Recently, Meier and Meier[9,10] demonstrated that a double row of anchors with linking sutures not only increased the size of the cuff repair footprint but also the pullout strength at the tuberosity. The clinical effectiveness of double-row techniques is still under investigation.

Increasing the number of anchors has a potential negative effect, however. As more anchors are inserted, the integrity of the remaining tuberosity may be compromised, weakening the hold of previously placed anchors. Multiple bioabsorbable anchors would theoretically increase the biologic load but could weaken the strength of the tuberosity. When the integrity of the tuberosity is severely compromised by osteopenia or cyst formation, alternative strategies for fixation are indicated, including placing suture anchors farther down the humeral shaft, using sutures in a tension-band mode, or converting to a mini-open approach using bone tunnels.

Suturing Technique

Arthroscopic rotator cuff repairs most commonly fail at the tendon-suture interface. Multiple stitch configurations have been described and tested in an attempt to maximize suture holding power in the tendon.[11-13]

An arthroscopic Mason-Allen equivalent stitch consists of a doubly loaded suture anchor with one stitch passed in a mattress fashion and the second passed over the first in simple fashion. A variety of double-row crossing patterns and tendon-holding suture techniques have been described, although no "best" pattern has been identified (**Figure 5**).[14]

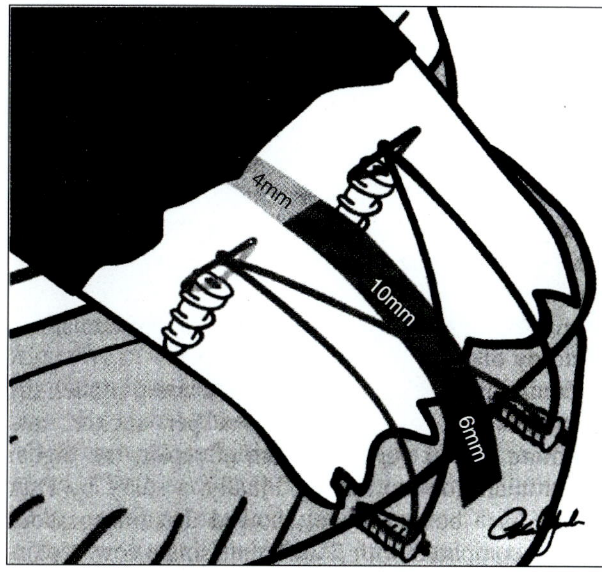

Figure 5 Double-row rotator cuff repair. (*Reproduced with permission from Cole BJ, ElAttrache NS, Anbari A: Arthroscopic rotator cuff repairs: An anatomic and biomechanical rationale for different suture-anchor repair configurations.* Arthroscopy *2007;23:662-669.*)

Reducing Tension on the Repair

A critical factor in rotator cuff repair is the tension at the repair site. Excessive tension at the site of a rotator cuff repair can be its undoing. Careful mobilization and lysis of adhesions and application of the principles of open rotator cuff repair are important in arthroscopic repair. Radiofrequency devices should be used to release adhesions while maintaining hemostasis. Intra-articular and extra-articular release will increase tendon excursion and decrease tension at the repair site. The surgeon can assess tension by using a traction stitch or tendon-holding clamp. The cuff tendon should be mobile enough to reach the lateral edge of the greater tuberosity.

Case Management and Outcome Summary

The patient's MRI scans revealed failure of the rotator cuff repair, without anchor pullout into the subacromial space. Laboratory studies were within normal limits. The patient required arthroscopic revision.

In the revision surgery, the sutures had pulled through the cuff tendon and were removed from the anchors. The rotator cuff was mobilized. Because the bone quality of the greater tuberosity appeared to be somewhat compromised after use of bioabsorbable sutures, a mini-open repair using bone tunnels was performed. The postoperative course was uneventful, and the patient returned to all her normal preoperative activities within 6 months.

Case Presentation

Case 2

A 65-year-old-man presented with ecchymosis in his left upper arm after injuring it in a fall. The patient had no history of prior shoulder problems, and his health was generally good. On physical examination, there was no evidence of shoulder atrophy or asymmetry, and his neck moved freely. Deltoid function and neurovascular examination findings were normal. Passive shoulder range of motion included forward flexion to 150°, external rotation to 50°, and internal rotation to the sacrum. Active elevation was limited to 130° because of pain, and there was marked weakness with external rotation.

Plain radiographs revealed no evidence of fracture, but some degenerative changes were seen at the acromioclavicular (AC) joint, with inferior spurring and a type 2 acromion. MRI of the shoulder revealed a full-thickness rotator cuff tear (**Figure 6**).

The patient underwent an arthroscopic acromioplasty, distal clavicle excision, and rotator cuff repair using a bioabsorbable anchor and bioabsorbable tack. Postoperatively, he continued to have pain and weakness and could not actively elevate his arm above shoulder level.

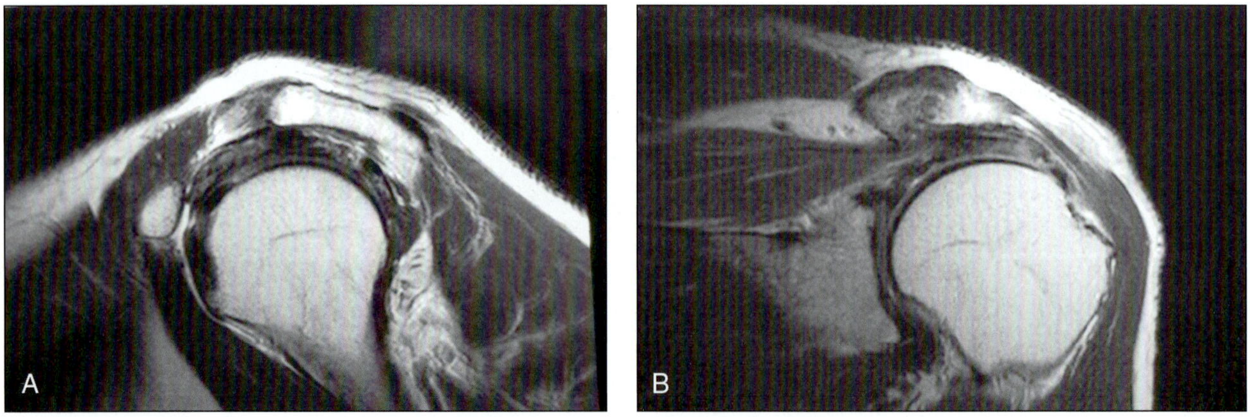

Figure 6 Preoperative MRI evaluation. T2-weighted MRI scans showing rotator cuff tearing and acromial contour.

Current Problem and Treatment

The patient had persistent, severe pain postoperatively and believed that his functioning had worsened. He had increasing difficulty sleeping and with activities of daily living and was unable to work.

Three months postoperatively, physical examination revealed moderate diffuse atrophy of the shoulder musculature. The deltoid appeared to be functioning, but there was a small area of detachment visible in the anterior third. His passive range of motion remained unchanged, but active elevation was now limited to only 60°. There was visible anterosuperior subluxation of the humeral head with any attempt at elevation and marked weakness of external rotation.

Axillary nerve sensation was intact, and the findings of the distal neurovascular examination were normal. Electromyography was positive for decreased conduction of the suprascapular nerve. Laboratory studies, including a complete blood cell count, C-reactive protein level, and erythrocyte sedimentation rate, were within normal limits.
Radiographs showed anterosuperior subluxation of the humeral head, and absence of the anterior half of the acromion was noted on a scapular-Y view (**Figure** 7). Repeat MRI revealed retraction and severe atrophy with fatty infiltration of the supraspinatus and infraspinatus muscles (**Figure** 8). Significant cartilage degeneration also was noted. After a lengthy discussion with the patient to review the available surgical options, a reverse shoulder arthroplasty was chosen.

Discussion

Recognizing the Problem

This patient had a failed rotator cuff repair with several compounding factors. The postoperative examination suggested anterosuperior escape of the humeral head caused by the loss of the coracoacromial arch in a rotator cuff-insufficient shoulder. Postoperative radiographs and MRI scans confirmed excessive acromioplasty and distal clavicle excision, with superior escape of the humeral head, deltoid detachment, and a rotator cuff tear. This combination of problems is one of the more severe complications associated with any rotator cuff tear repair.

Role of Acromioplasty

The need for acromioplasty when repairing a rotator cuff tear has been challenged by several authors.[15,16] In patients with an acute rotator cuff tear and no previous rotator cuff symptoms, the need for acromioplasty and AC joint excision should be carefully assessed. In these patients, bursal excision and rotator cuff repair may be sufficient.

When performing acromioplasty, the amount of acromial bone to be removed should be carefully determined during preoperative evaluation. In patients with large rotator cuff tears, excessive acromioplasty increases the risk for anterosuperior humeral subluxation if the cuff repair fails, with pseudoparalysis as an unfortunate result. Excessive acromioplasty can also lead to loss or weakening of

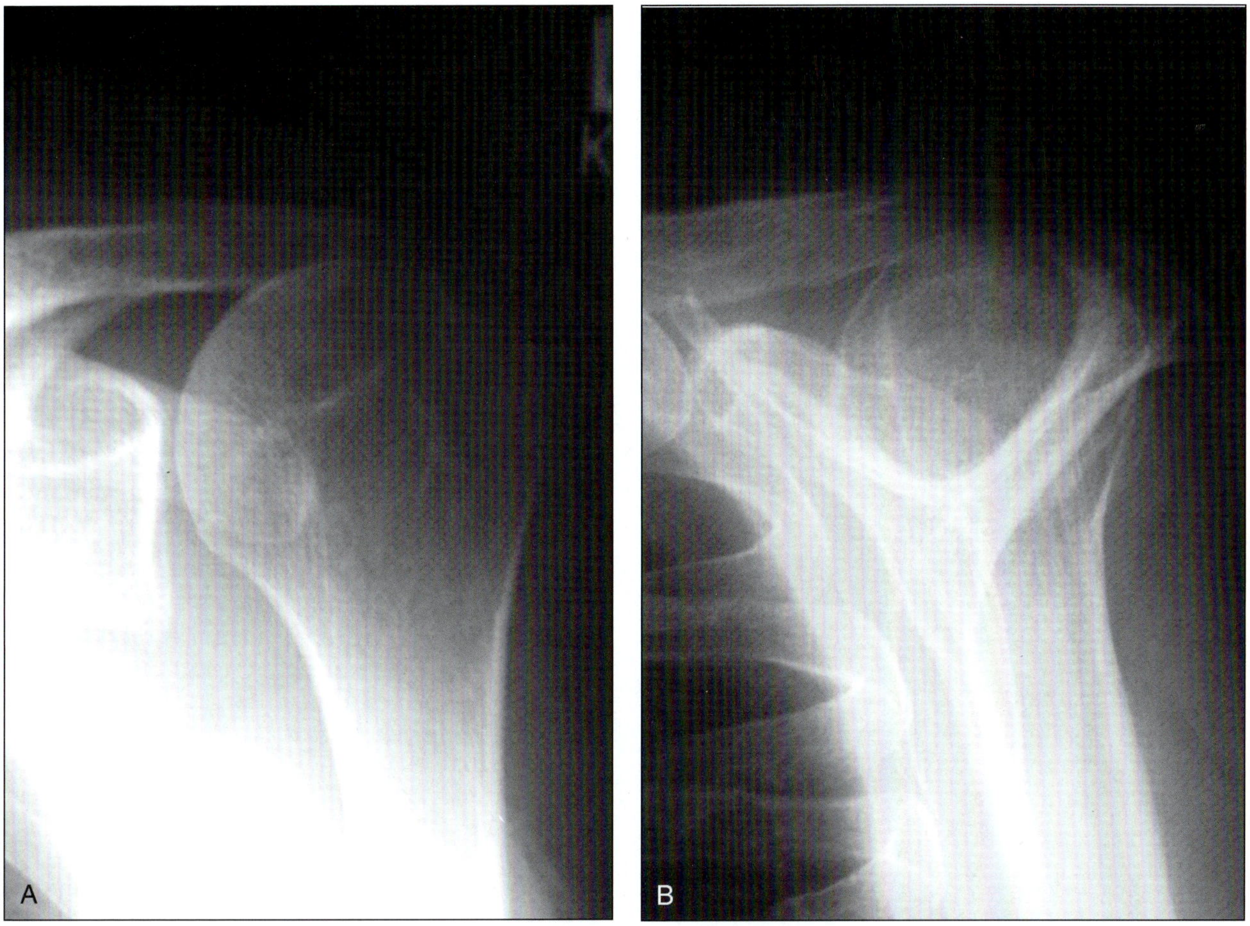

Figure 7 Postoperative radiographs reveal superior migration of the humeral head and acromial resection.

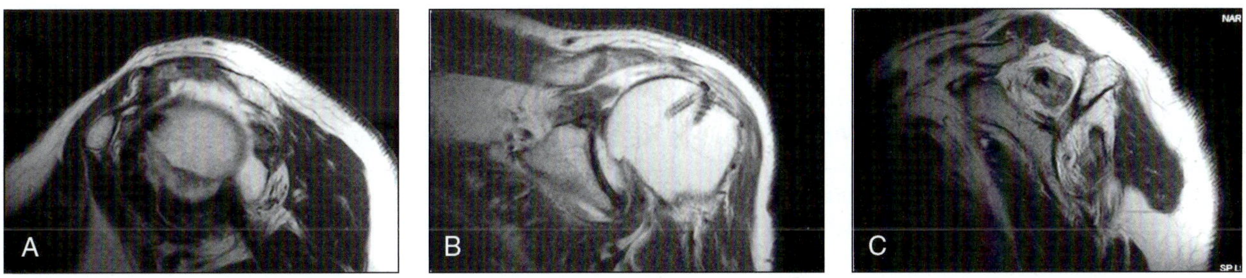

Figure 8 Postoperative MRI scans reveal the extent of acromial resection, failure of the cuff repair, and marked atrophy and fatty infiltration of retracted cuff tissue.

the deltoid origin, which could potentially compromise any salvage procedure, such as a latissimus dorsi muscle transfer or a reverse shoulder arthroplasty.

Suprascapular Nerve Injury

The patient's postoperative MRI scans showed severe atrophy and fatty infiltration of both the supraspinatus

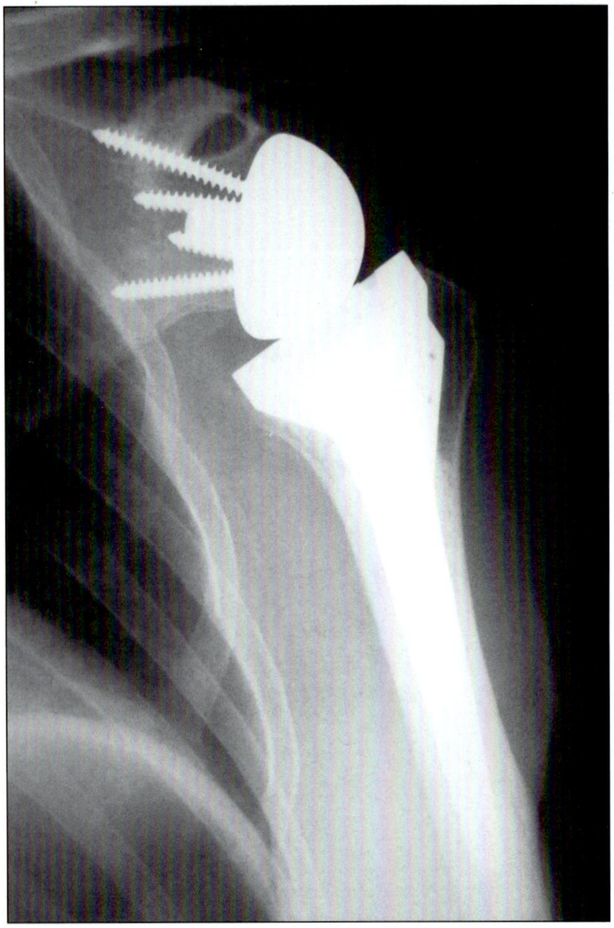

Figure 9 Reverse shoulder arthroplasty.

and infraspinatus muscles. Suprascapular nerve palsy may accompany large rotator cuff tears[17] and can contribute to failure of cuff repair as the humeral head translates superiorly with deltoid contraction in the absence of the rotator cuff acting as a fulcrum. Contact between the cuff and coracoacromial arch is inevitable, and mechanical stresses make cuff healing difficult.

The etiology of suprascapular nerve palsy is not clear but may be the result of traction on the nerve as the rotator cuff retracts medially. Restoring cuff integrity and length may allow for nerve recovery in some patients.

Direct injury to the suprascapular nerve during cuff mobilization also may occur. Cadaveric studies have demonstrated that the suprascapular nerve traverses the suprascapular notch at a distance of 2.9 ± 0.3 cm from the glenoid rim.[18] Furthermore, the distance from the glenoid rim to the nerve at the spine of the scapula is only 1.8 ± 0.2 cm. The relative proximity of the suprascapular nerve to these bony structures places the nerve at risk during intra-articular mobilization of the cuff; therefore, care should be taken when adhesions are released beyond 1.4-cm from the glenoid rim posteriorly.

Management of the Problem

Several compounding factors make management of this combination of complications difficult. Deltoid detachment with subsequent repair often is associated with poor results, suprascapular nerve palsy will complicate any attempt at repair, and severe atrophy with fatty infiltration makes primary repair unlikely to succeed or to restore function.[19]

Latissimus dorsi transfer could be considered in combination with deltoid repair, but early degenerative changes on MRI scans with significant pain in an older patient makes this a less attractive option. Reverse shoulder arthroplasty could be considered as well, but the results can be compromised by an abnormal anterior deltoid. In patients younger than 70 years, inevitable problems associated with reverse shoulder replacement include wearing, loosening, and the need for revision surgery. No simple solution exists for this patient; therefore, prevention of this combination of complications should be paramount.

Case Management and Outcome Summary

The patient continued to have severe pain and pseudoparalysis with nonsurgical management. He opted for reverse shoulder arthroplasty after an extensive review of the surgical options, which included latissimus dorsi muscle transfer and deltoid repair. Despite his relatively young age, reverse shoulder arthroplasty (**Figure 9**) was performed, with attempted repair of the deltoid detachment. Postoperatively, good pain relief was achieved, and he could actively elevate his arm to 120°; however, his strength remained compromised by the partial deltoid detachment. He was happy with the pain relief but disappointed in the functional result.

Strategies to Minimize Common Complications

Failure of rotator cuff repair is multifactorial. Failure can occur because of intrinsic cuff tissue problems (poor tissue quality, inelasticity, or scarring), insufficient healing (compliance issues, overly aggressive physical therapy, obesity, smoking), or failure of fixation (suture breakage or pull through, anchor pullout, inadequate repair).

Rotator cuff repair is most often successful with good visualization and understanding of the tear pattern. Mobilization of the cuff is essential for a tension-free repair. Suture anchor placement must be appropriate for the tear pattern, and anchors should be tested for pullout strength prior to repair. Visualization from the lateral portal allows the best appreciation of the tear pattern. Crescent-shaped tears may be repaired directly to bone, but L-shaped or U-shaped configurations may require tendon-to-tendon suturing to improve repair integrity and fixation. Margin convergence of U-shaped tears can be helpful in closing very large, retracted tears prior to tuberosity fixation. The various configurations of anchor placement and suture passage that have been reported are still being debated; however, larger tears generally require more anchors spaced evenly across the tuberosity.

Successful arthroscopic rotator cuff repair also relies on appropriate postoperative management. Most authors agree that active motion should be delayed approximately 4 to 6 weeks after surgery to allow for initial cuff healing, but no consensus exists on the optimum postoperative regimen. Postoperative exercise programs should progress according to surgeon-assessed factors, such as tear size, repair type, tendon involvement, and tendon quality. Resistive exercises are limited for 8 to 12 weeks, again depending on the security of the repair. Patients should be advised preoperatively of the importance of closely following postoperative protocols. The absence of significant pain after arthroscopic repair can be misleading to patients who may attempt vigorous exercise too quickly.

Finally, successful arthroscopic rotator cuff repair requires the surgeon to be skilled in many aspects of arthroscopic surgery. The ability to visualize and recognize the pathology and then conceptualize the steps needed for repair is critical. The skills for performing each step of surgery, including acromioplasty, distal clavicle excision, cuff mobilization, anchor placement, suture management, and knot tying, need to be present and well honed for successful arthroscopic repair. Each portion of the repair should be done quickly to avoid excessive tissue edema, which will make each subsequent portion of the surgery more challenging. Skilled arthroscopists can generally perform an acromioplasty or distal clavicle excision in 10 to 20 minutes. The surgeon who does not possess these skills should consider open or mini-open repair, which have been successful for a great number of patients.

References

1. Brislin KJ, Field LD, Savoie FH: Complications after arthroscopic rotator cuff repair. *Arthroscopy* 2007;23:124-128.
2. Athwal GS, Sperling JW, Rispoli DM, Cofield RH: Deep infection after rotator cuff repair. *J Shoulder Elbow Surg* 2007;16:306-311.
3. Burkart A, Imhoff AB, Roscher E: Foreign-body reaction to the bioabsorbable suretac device. *Arthroscopy* 2000;16:91-95.
4. Tingart MJ, Apreleva M, Lehtinen J, Zurakowski D, Warner JJ: Anchor design and bone mineral density affect the pull-out strength of suture anchors in rotator cuff repair: Which anchors are best to use in patients with low bone quality? *Am J Sports Med* 2004;32:1466-1473.
5. Burkhart SS, Klein JR: Arthroscopic repair of rotator cuff tears associated with large bone cysts of the proximal humerus: Compaction bone grafting technique. *Arthroscopy* 2005;21:1149.
6. Tingart MJ, Apreleva M, Zurakowski D, Warner JJ: Pullout strength of suture anchors used in rotator cuff repair. *J Bone Joint Surg Am* 2003;85:2190-2198.
7. Brady PC, Arrigoni P, Burkhart SS: What do you do when you have a loose screw? *Arthroscopy* 2006;22:925-930.
8. Liporace FA, Bono CM, Caruso SA, Weiner B, Penny K, Feldman AJ, Grossman MG, Haher TR: The mechanical effects of suture anchor insertion angle for rotator cuff repair. *Orthopedics* 2002;25:399-402.
9. Meier SW, Meier JD: Rotator cuff repair: The effect of double-row fixation on three-dimensional repair site. *J Shoulder Elbow Surg* 2006;15:691-696.

10. Meier SW, Meier JD: The effect of double-row fixation on initial repair strength in rotator cuff repair: A biomechanical study. *Arthroscopy* 2006;22:1168-1173.
11. Macgillivray JD, Ma CB: An arthroscopic stitch for massive rotator cuff tears: The Mac stitch. *Arthroscopy* 2004;20:669-671.
12. Ma CB, Macgillivray JD, Clabeaux J, Lee S, Otis JC: Biomechanical evaluation of arthroscopic rotator cuff stitches. *J Bone Joint Surg Am* 2004;86:1211-1216.
13. Castagna A, Garafolo R, Conti M, Borroni M, Snyder SJ: Arthroscopic rotator cuff repair using a triple-loaded suture anchor and a modified Mason-Allen technique (Alex stitch). *Arthroscopy* 2007;23:440.e1-4.
14. Nho SJ, Yadav H, Pensak M, Dodson CC, Good CR, Macgillivray JD: Biomechanical fixation in arthroscopic rotator cuff repair. *Arthroscopy* 2007;23:94-102.
15. McCallister WV, Parsons IM, Titelman RM, Matsen FA: Open rotator cuff repair without acromioplasty. *J Bone Joint Surg Am* 2005;87:1278-1283.
16. Milano G, Grasso A, Salvatore M, Zarelli D, Deriu L, Fabbriciani C: Arthroscopic rotator cuff repair with and without subacromial decompression: A prospective randomized study. *Arthroscopy* 2007;23:81-88.
17. Mallon WJ, Wilson RJ, Basamania CJ: The association of suprascapular neuropathy with massive rotator cuff tears: A preliminary report. *J Shoulder Elbow Surg* 2006;15:395-398.
18. Shishido H, Kikuchi S: Injury of the suprascapular nerve in shoulder surgery: An anatomic study. *J Shoulder Elbow Surg* 2001;10:372-376.
19. Gerber C, Schneeberger AG, Hoppeler H, Meyer DC: Correlation of atrophy and fatty infiltration on strength and integrity of rotator cuff repairs: A study in thirteen patients. *J Shoulder Elbow Surg* 2007;16:691-696.

Chapter 5

Failed Subacromial Decompression

Donald P. Endrizzi, MD

Case Presentation

A 46-year-old, right-handed roofer presented with a 1-year history of pain in his right shoulder, particularly with overhead activities. The pain also occasionally awakened him from sleep. Over the past 6 months, the patient has followed a vigorous program of rotator cuff strengthening. He has tried several over-the-counter anti-inflammatory medications to control the pain and was given a subacromial cortisone injection, which provided a brief, 2-week period of pain relief.

On physical examination, the patient had full active and passive range of motion at the shoulder, but Neer and Hawkins impingement signs were positive. There was no acromioclavicular (AC) joint tenderness or prominence, and no evidence of instability. AP, scapular-Y, and axillary radiographs showed a prominence on the acromion, consistent with a type II (curved) acromial morphology. There was no prominence on the distal clavicle and no abnormalities in the glenohumeral joint. An MRI scan showed supraspinatus tendinopathy, but no evidence of rotator cuff tearing. A diagnostic subacromial cortisone injection was performed, and the patient had complete relief of pain on impingement testing.

Initial Surgery

The patient underwent arthroscopic subacromial decompression. Intra-articular inspection showed no abnormalities of the superior labrum, biceps tendon, rotator cuff, or glenohumeral joint; however, subacromial evaluation revealed thickened bursal tissue, visible fraying of the coracoacromial ligament on the undersurface of the acromion, and some minor fraying of the outer surface of the rotator cuff (**Figure 1**).

Soft tissue on the undersurface of the acromion was removed with an electrocautery wand, and a burr was used to remove bone from the anterior half of the acromion, tapering posteriorly. The patient had no postoperative complications; however, 6 months after surgery, the pathologic signs and symptoms were unchanged from his preoperative evaluation.

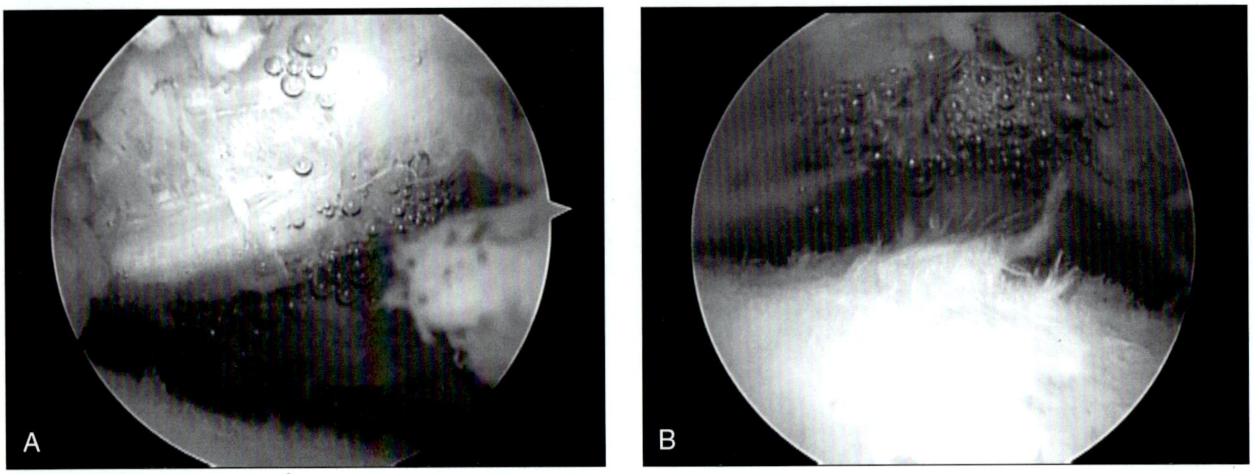

Figure 1 Arthroscopic images from the posterior viewing portal reveal fraying of the coracoacromial ligament **(A)** and the outer surface of the supraspinatus muscle **(B)**.

Table 1: Reasons for Failed Subacromial Decompression

Misdiagnosis
- Intra-articular pathology
    - Arthritis
    - Labral tears
- Nonoutlet Impingement
    - Posterior capsular tightness
    - Shoulder instability
    - Rotator cuff weakness
    - Scapular dysfunction
- Os acromiale
- Acromioclavicular arthrosis
    - AC joint pain
    - AC osteophytes

Surgical Errors or Complications
- Inadequate acromioplasty
- Excessive bone resection
    - Deltoid detachment
    - Anterosuperior instability
- Postoperative stiffness, adhesions

Discussion

Recognizing Failed Subacromial Decompression

This scenario highlights some of the potential pitfalls of subacromial decompression surgery. Since 1972, open acromioplasty, as described by Neer,[1] has become a widely accepted procedure in the treatment of shoulder impingement syndrome, with published success rates of 85% to 90%. Similar outcomes have been reported for arthroscopic subacromial decompression.[2,3]

Surgical failure may occur in several ways[4] (**Table 1**). Diagnostic errors are a common cause of failed acromioplasty. Posterior capsular tightness, instability, intra-articular pathology, and abnormal scapular mechanics all can mimic the symptoms of mechanical outlet impingement and can lead to surgical failure if not recognized. Additionally, concomitant pathology, such as AC joint arthritis, may exist.

Iatrogenic errors are another common cause of failed acromioplasty. Surgical technique and skills should be honed prior to any surgical procedure to provide consistent, reproducible results. With experience, complications of acromioplasty caused by poor technique, such as deltoid detachment, can be minimized.

Managing the Failed Acromioplasty

Management of a failed acromioplasty begins with reestablishing the diagnosis. Physical examination of the patient should reveal full range of motion at the shoulder, with little or no restriction of internal rotation. There should be no AC joint tenderness and no evidence of instability.

Radiographs should be obtained, including AP, scapular-Y, and axillary views, and should show ade-

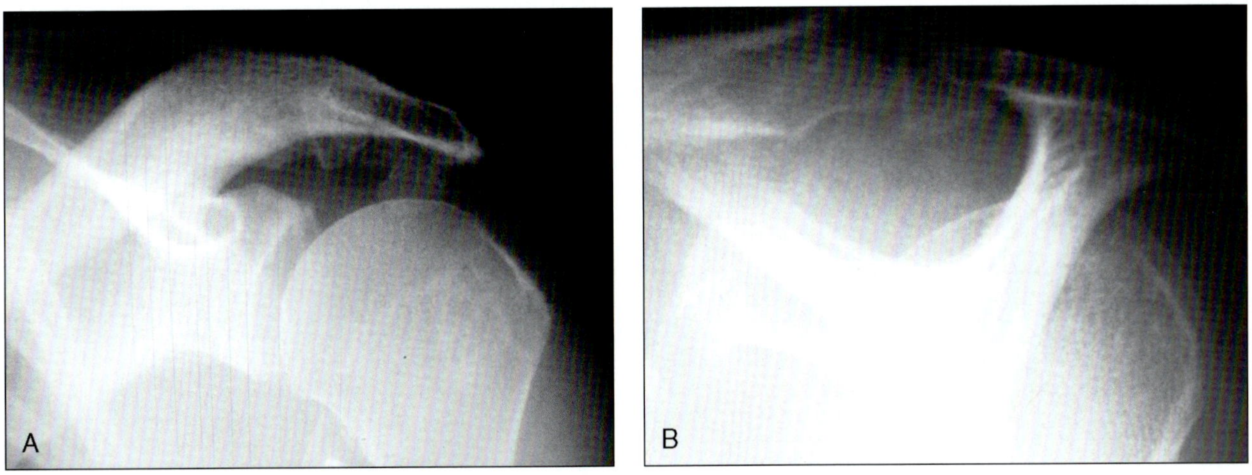

Figure 2 AP **(A)** and scapular-Y **(B)** radiographs show an acromial fracture post acromioplasty.

quate subacromial decompression with no other abnormalities, such as acromial fracture (**Figure 2**) or distal clavicular prominence.

A diagnostic subacromial cortisone injection should be given. If this test is equivocal, further evaluation with MRI might be helpful to look for other sources of pathology.

Preventing Failed Acromioplasty

Establishing the Correct Diagnosis

Weber[5] noted that most patients needing revision acromioplasty were initially operated on for the wrong diagnosis. To avoid or minimize diagnostic errors, a subacromial injection test, as described by Neer,[1] should be performed prior to acromioplasty to confirm the diagnosis of impingement and to rule out other sources of shoulder pain. Relief of symptoms over several days or weeks after a corticosteroid injection does not in itself establish the diagnosis of impingement, however, because cortisone, through its anti-inflammatory effect, may relieve discomfort from various sources. Nevertheless, the importance of a positive subacromial injection test in patients with shoulder impingement cannot be underestimated.[6,7]

Other causes of shoulder pain, such as postoperative stiffness or instability, should be excluded prior to surgery through the patient history, physical examination, and appropriate imaging studies. Posterior capsular tightness can cause impingement that will not be addressed by acromioplasty. Young athletes with symptoms of impingement should be carefully assessed for subtle instability as a cause of rotator cuff tendinitis. Abnormalities in scapular mechanics or winging might also contribute to impingement symptoms. Intra-articular pathology, such as an osteochondral injury or labral tear, should be considered if subacromial injection fails to provide pain relief.

Adequate Bone Resection

Insufficient bone resection is a common cause of persistent symptoms following acromioplasty. Simply removing a standard amount of bone (ie, 5 mm) may be adequate for some patients but inadequate for larger patients or those with extensive calcification of the coracoacromial ligament (**Figure 3**). Conversely, removal of 5 mm of bone may be excessive in smaller patients and may lead to detachment of the deltoid.[8]

Failure to appreciate bone spurring in the AC joint as a cause of impingement can also leave a patient with residual symptoms. Preoperative radiographs can be used to estimate the amount of acromial resection needed. The supraspinatus outlet view, which provides a lateral view of the acromion, is useful for this and for visualizing osteophytes in the AC joint. An axillary radiograph may show the presence of an

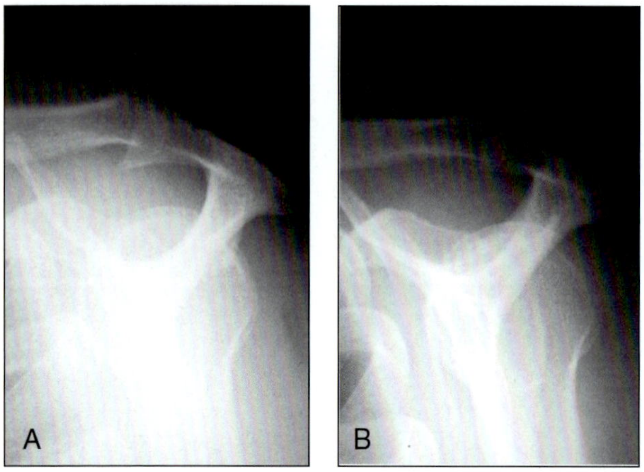

Figure 3 Preoperative **(A)** and postoperative **(B)** outlet radiographs show a successful acromioplasty.

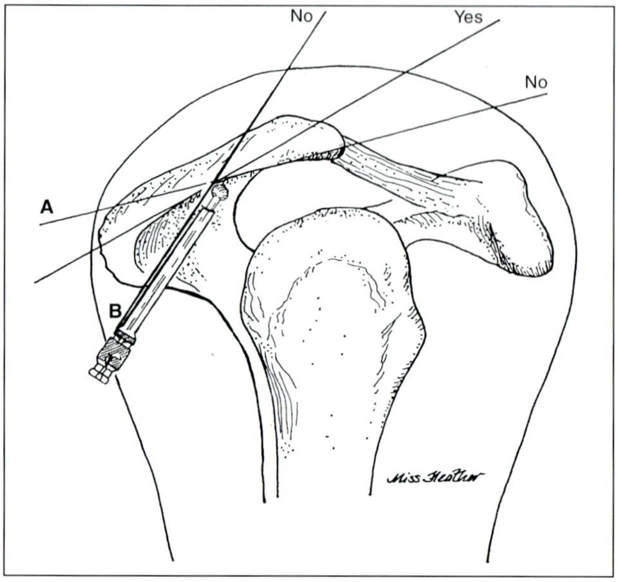

Figure 4 The effect of portal placement on the cutting-block technique. Portal placement too high posteriorly **(A)** may result in insufficient acromial resection, whereas an inferiorly placed portal **(B)** may result in excessive resection. (*Reproduced with permission from Caspari RB, Thal R: A technique for arthroscopic subacromial decompression.* Arthroscopy *1992;8:23-30.*)

os acromiale, which may change the surgical approach or the amount of acromial resection. A small acromial ossicle may be resected completely, but resection of a large acromial fragment may risk detachment of the deltoid. Open reduction and internal fixation should be considered for the patient with a large, painful, os acromiale. AC joint resection in association with an os acromiale may create instability and pain in patients with a previously painless acromion, requiring subsequent open reduction and internal fixation.

During arthroscopy, the acromial burr diameter can be used to gauge the amount of bone resection. Ellman[9] suggested creating a trough of known depth along the anterior acromial undersurface and then tapering the remaining acromion posteriorly from that trough. He used a posterior viewing portal and a lateral resection portal. The lateral portal should be placed about 3 cm distal to the lateral acromial border, low enough for the shaver to be effective on the anteromedial acromion.

The cutting-block technique, performed with the arthroscope in the lateral portal and the arthroscopic burr in the posterior portal, is used by some surgeons to reliably resect an adequate amount of bone.[10] Proper portal placement with the cutting-block technique is critical (**Figure 4**). The posterior portal should be 2 cm to 3 cm distal to the posterior acromion. Portal placement too high posteriorly may result in insufficient acromial resection; placement too low may result in excessive resection.

Establishing Clear Visualization and Orientation

Regardless of technique, clear visualization and orientation in the subacromial space is essential to avoid complications. Resection of the subacromial bursa will allow for visualization of the entire subacromial space and rotator cuff.

The anterior and lateral edges of the acromion must be clearly delineated intraoperatively. If there is confusion intraoperatively regarding the subacromial landmarks, placement of needle or suture markers at the anteromedial and anterolateral borders of the acromion may serve to reorient the surgeon (**Figure 5**).

The surgeon should be constantly aware of the orientation of the acromion and should maintain camera position with respect to acromial orientation. Occasionally, when the edges of the acromion are not well defined, the surgeon may inadvertently remove bone from the center of the acromion and fail to remove bone from the anteromedial or anterolateral acromial borders, which can put the acromion at risk for fracture but not address the offending bony prominence. If it becomes difficult to assess the adequacy of acromial resection because of fluid extravasation, bleeding, or other technical problems, a direct digital palpation of the acromion can be performed through a slightly enlarged lateral portal, as suggested by Hawkins and associates.[11]

Disorientation within the subacromial space may also lead to excessive bone resection at the lateral or anterior borders of the acromion, with detachment of the deltoid as an unfortunate result. An os acromiale can lead to confusion intraoperatively and can be mistaken for the AC joint if not identified on preoperative imaging. Removal of soft tissue from the anterior half of the acromial undersurface should be complete enough to allow visualization of the anterior and lateral borders. Deltoid fibers will be seen during resection and should alert the surgeon as to the adequacy of resection.

Poor hemostasis can also lead to inadequate visualization. Electrocautery is required to control bleeding from the acromial branch of the thoracoacromial artery. Hypotensive anesthesia can be helpful but should be used carefully in older patients or those with atherosclerotic cardiovascular disease. Maintenance of adequate fluid pressure will aid in the control of bleeding, but can quickly lead to extravasation of fluid if pump pressure is high.

Clearly defining the anterior and lateral borders of the acromion by clearing soft tissue and maintaining camera orientation can help the surgeon avoid excessive or misdirected resection. When deltoid fibers are seen at the acromial edge, the surgeon should stop and assess burr position, orientation, and the need for further bone resection. Heterotopic ossification with recurrent impingement[12] and loss of deltoid function[13] has been reported after acromioplasty, but is rare.

Case Management and Outcome Summary

The history and radiographs in this patient suggest a failed acromioplasty. Physical examination revealed findings that were unchanged from the preoperative evaluation: full active and passive shoulder range of motion, positive impingement signs, and no AC joint tenderness. The postoperative radiographs showed an inadequate acromioplasty, with removal of the anteromedial acromial undersurface but leaving the anterolateral portion (**Figure 6**). A repeat corticosteroid injection test completely relieved the patient's symptoms.

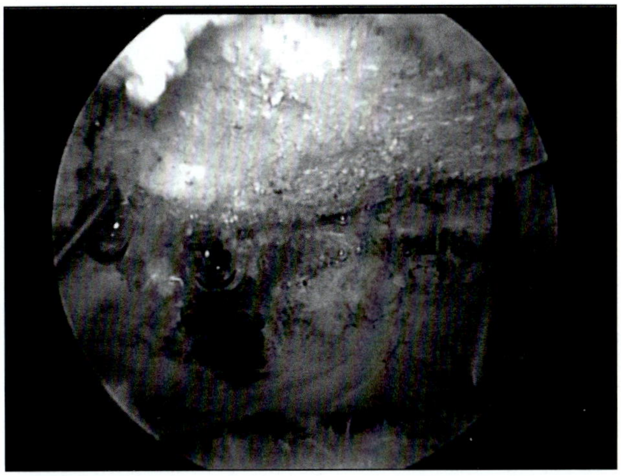

Figure 5 Arthroscopic image shows placement of needle markers at the anteromedial and anterolateral borders of the acromion.

Findings from the initial arthroscopic surgery failed to demonstrate additional intra-articular pathology. The patient was returned to the operating room for diagnostic arthroscopy and revision acromioplasty. A prominent acromion and frayed coracoacromial ligament fibers were noted anteromedially, and the acromioplasty and coracoacromial ligament release were revised. Twelve weeks after revision surgery, the patient was asymptomatic and able to return to all of his preoperative activities.

Strategies to Minimize Common Complications

The diagnosis of outlet impingement should be firmly established prior to acromioplasty. Other causes of shoulder pain should be considered and evaluated to avoid diagnostic errors. Nonoutlet impingement, os acromiale, AC joint involvement, and intra-articular pathology should be identified when present to avoid unsuccessful acromioplasty.

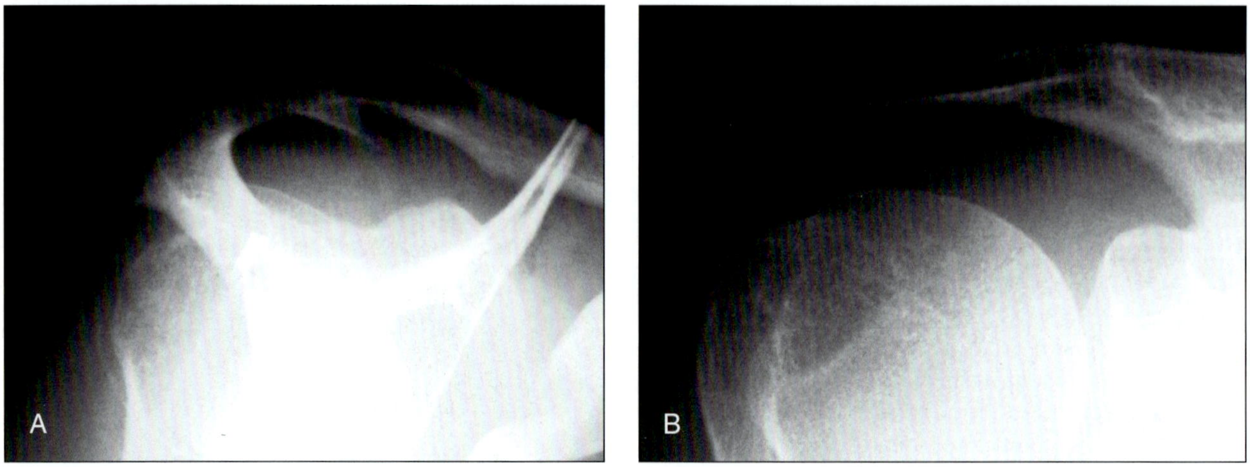

Figure 6 Postoperative radiographs revealing inadequate acromioplasty with anteromedial resection.

Arthroscopic technique should be mastered prior to surgery. Maintaining orientation within the subacromial space, providing clear visualization of landmarks, and resecting an appropriate amount of bone will help minimize technical failures of arthroscopic acromioplasty.

REFERENCES

1. Neer CS: Anterior acromioplasty for chronic impingement syndrome in the shoulder: A preliminary report. *J Bone Joint Surg Am* 1972;54:45-51.
2. Spangehl MJ, Hawkins RH, McCormack RG, Loomer RL: Arthroscopic versus open acromioplasty: A prospective, randomized, blinded study. *J Shoulder Elbow Surg* 2002;11:101-107.
3. Barfield LC, Kuhn JE: Arthroscopic versus open acromioplasty: A systematic review. *Clin Orthop Relat Res* 2007;455:64-71.
4. Ogilvie-Harris DJ, Wiley AM, Sattarian J: Failed acromioplasty for impingement syndrome. *J Bone Joint Surg Br* 1990;72:1070-1072.
5. Weber SC: Revision arthroscopy: An arthroscopic approach. *Orthop Trans* 1996;20:919.
6. Mair SD, Viola RW, Gill TJ, Briggs KK, Hawkins RJ: Can the impingement test predict outcome after arthroscopic subacromial decompression? *J Shoulder Elbow Surg* 2004;13:150-153.
7. Lim JT, Acornley A, Dodenhoff RM: Recovery after arthroscopic subacromial decompression: Prognostic value of the subacromial injection test. *Arthroscopy* 2005;21:680-683.
8. Green A, Griggs S, Labrador D: Anterior acromial anatomy: Relevance to arthroscopic acromioplasty. *Arthroscopy* 2004;20:1050-1054.
9. Ellman H: Arthroscopic subacromial decompression: Analysis of one- to three-year results. *Arthroscopy* 1987;3:173-181.
10. Caspari RB, Thal R: A technique for arthroscopic subacromial decompression. *Arthroscopy* 1992;8:23-30.
11. Hawkins RJ, Plancher KD, Saddemi SR, Brezenoff LS, Moor JT: Arthroscopic subacromial decompression. *J Shoulder Elbow Surg* 2001;10:225-230.
12. Berg EE, Ciullo JV, Ogelsby JW: Failure of arthroscopic decompression by subacromial heterotopic ossification causing recurrent impingement. *Arthroscopy* 1994;10:158-161.
13. Boynton MD, Enders TJ: Severe heterotopic ossification after arthroscopic acromioplasty: A case report. *J Shoulder Elbow Surg* 1999;8:495-497.

Chapter 6

Inadequate Acromioclavicular Joint Resection

Donald P. Endrizzi, MD

Case Presentation

A 50-year-old, right-handed orthopaedic surgeon presented with a 5-year history of intermittent right shoulder pain localized to the acromioclavicular (AC) joint. He has pain with activities of daily living and is often awakened at night by shoulder pain. An avid skier, he gave a history of a number of minor injuries to his AC joint. Over the past year, the patient has received several injections of local anesthetic into the joint, providing good short-term pain relief; however, after each injection there was a recurrence of pain within 2 to 6 weeks.

On physical examination, the patient had normal cervical spine motion and full active and passive range of motion of the shoulder. Pain was elicited on palpation of the AC joint and during cross-chest compression and internal rotation of the shoulder. The O'Brien test was negative, as were impingement signs. A diagnostic injection of 1% lidocaine into the AC joint provided complete relief of his symptoms.

Plain radiographs revealed narrowing of the AC joint, with periarticular cysts and inferior osteophyte formation (**Figure 1**). Mild indentation of the rotator cuff was visible on MRI scans. The glenohumeral joint appeared normal, without labral pathology.

Initial Surgery

Intra-articular inspection of the glenohumeral joint revealed no abnormalities, and the patient underwent arthroscopic AC joint excision via an inferior approach, with visualization through the subacromial space. The posterior subacromial portal was used as the viewing portal throughout the procedure. Inferior osteophytes were resected from the distal clavicle and acromion through a lateral portal, and distal clavicle excision was performed through an anterior portal aligned with the AC joint. A minimal acromioplasty was performed, primarily to provide complete visualization of the AC joint.

The patient began pendulum exercises on postoperative day 1 and progressed to activities of daily living as tolerated.

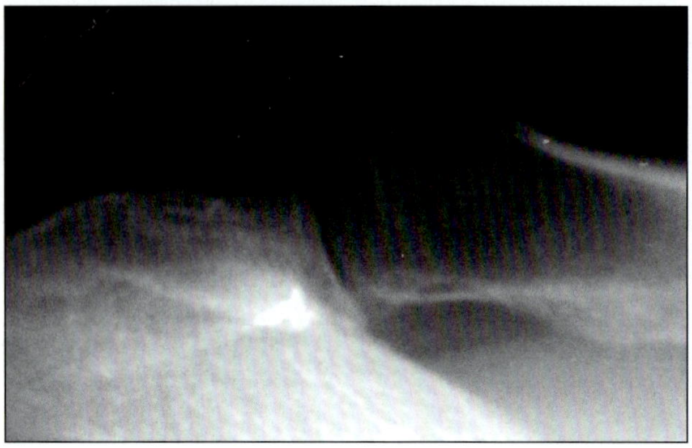

Figure 1 Preoperative radiograph reveals joint-space narrowing, cyst formation, and inferior osteophytes in the AC joint.

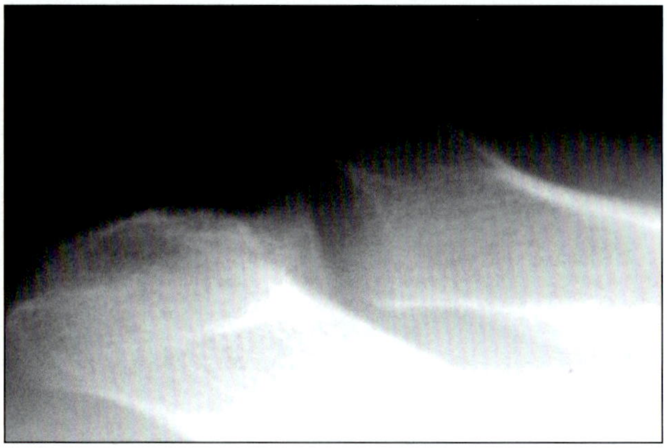

Figure 2 Postoperative radiograph shows inadequate superior resection of the distal clavicle.

Current Problem and Treatment

The patient continued to have pain and occasional snapping at the AC joint 6 months after surgery. Physical examination revealed full active and passive shoulder range of motion, but there was persistent pain and tenderness at the distal clavicle.

Postoperative radiographs demonstrated significant bone remaining at the superior aspect of the distal clavicle, suggestive of an inadequately resected AC joint (**Figure 2**). Injection of 2 mL of 1% lidocaine at the AC joint provided complete relief of symptoms, and the patient was recommended for revision arthroscopic AC joint resection.

Discussion

Recognizing the Problem

Pain following distal clavicle excision can be the result of a number of factors, including misdiagnosis, AC instability, and insufficient resection. Management of persistent pain following AC resection should begin with a thorough reevaluation of the patient.

A careful review of the patient history, physical examination findings, and radiographs is needed to isolate the cause of residual discomfort. Pain from cervical spine pathology may refer to the trapezius and the region of the AC joint; therefore, a neck examination should be part of the evaluation of a failed AC joint resection. Patients with superior labrum anterior to posterior (SLAP) lesions may present with shoulder pain and tenderness that can be mistaken for AC pathology; therefore, O'Brien and Speed tests should be included in the physical examination. Spinoglenoid cysts associated with labral tears also may be a source of pain. Strength testing may reveal rotational weakness. Patients may also have coexisting impingement from acromial osteophytes or from morphology not addressed completely by distal clavicle excision.

Selective injection of the AC joint with local anesthetic is often helpful in confirming the AC joint as the source of pain. Care should be taken during this procedure so that the needle remains within the joint and does not penetrate into the subacromial space, which may result in masking of the underlying subacromial pathology. Unfortunately, diagnostic injection in patients who have previously undergone inferior resection is somewhat unreliable, because the inferior capsule is no longer there to prevent infiltration into the subacromial space and may yield a false positive result in a patient with residual impingement.

Plain radiographs may reveal an inadequate resection, with bone remaining at the posterosuperior aspect of the distal clavicle, or they may show an overly aggressive resection, with resultant AC instability (**Figure 3**). MRI scans may show degenerative changes, even in patients without significant AC joint symptoms, and therefore should be viewed in conjunction with physical findings. Bone edema on MRI scan is sugges-

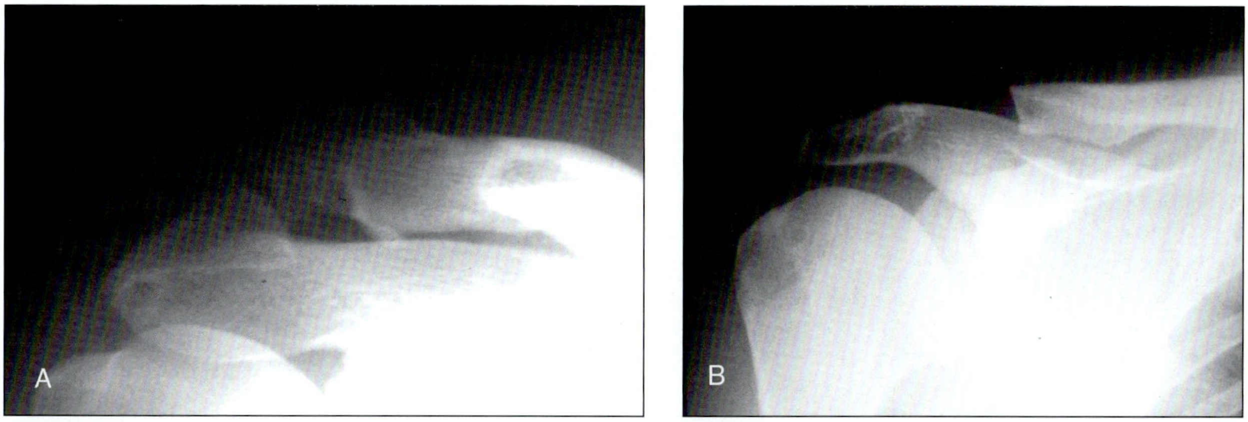

Figure 3 A, Inadequate resection of posterosuperior bone. **B,** Aggressive resection of the clavicle may lead to anterior-posterior instability.

tive of AC joint disease but does not confirm the AC joint as the definitive source of symptoms. MRI is often helpful in demonstrating other sources of shoulder pathology if symptoms are not limited to the AC joint.

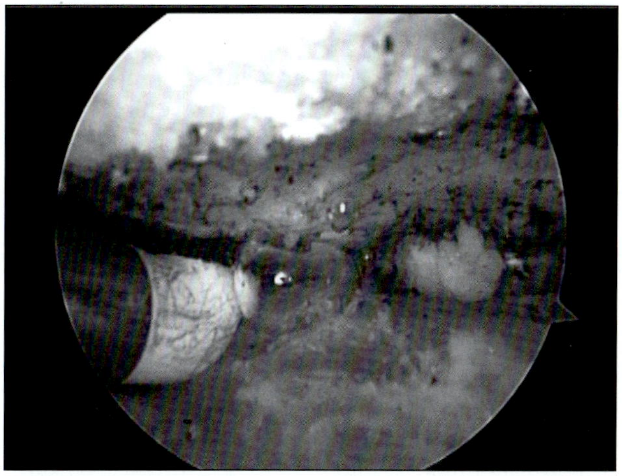

Figure 4 Exposure of the inferior clavicle using a posterior viewing portal and a lateral working portal. Cautery is used to control bleeding.

Techniques of AC Joint Excision

AC joint resection can be effectively performed through a direct approach into the joint or indirectly through the subacromial space.[1] With either approach, complete visualization of the distal clavicle is necessary to ensure proper resection.

Indirect Approach

The indirect (subacromial) approach is most commonly used for distal clavicle excision. In this technique, a posterior portal is established for viewing and a lateral working portal is created initially. Bursa and soft tissue are removed from the subacromial space to maximize visualization of the undersurface of the AC joint (**Figure 4**). Bleeding occurs frequently in the fatty tissues beneath the joint; therefore, most soft-tissue resection is done using ablative cautery throughout the procedure. The inferior capsule is removed with a soft-tissue ablator, but the posterior capsule is left intact. Inferior osteophytes are resected from the acromial facet and distal clavicle, allowing clear viewing into the AC joint from below (**Figure 5**).

An anterior portal is then established in line with the AC joint for direct débridement of soft tissue and bone. (Nonlinear portal placement with respect to the AC joint can make resection difficult or impossible.) When AC joint resection is planned as part of another procedure, such as rotator cuff repair, portal placement should be considered when initial portals are established. Skin marking at the beginning of the procedure, before any soft-tissue swelling occurs, can be helpful. A spinal needle can be helpful in confirming portal placement in obese patients. After clearing the subacromial space, the needle can be passed under direct visualization beneath and in line with the AC joint to guide portal placement (**Figure 6**).

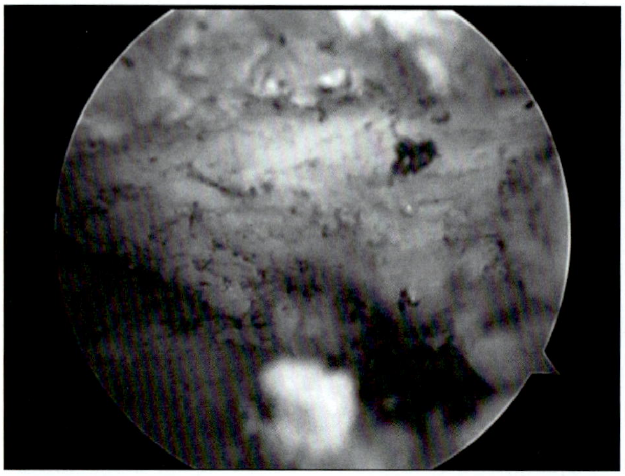

Figure 5 Visualization of the distal clavicle from the posterior portal.

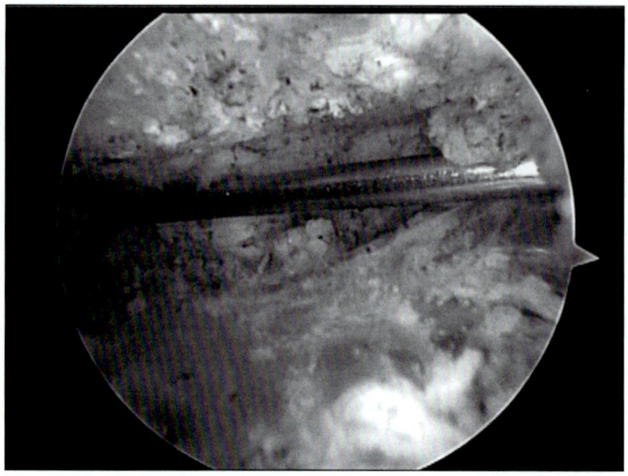

Figure 6 Spinal needle localization to guide placement of an anterior portal for distal clavicle resection.

Resection is performed through the anterior portal until the appropriate amount of bone is removed and visualization of the distal clavicle is clear. The burr is used as a guide to gauge the amount of bone resection. Bone resection can proceed in small increments using a sweeping technique across the face of the clavicle in order to remove bone evenly. Several passes, taking 1 mm to 3 mm of bone with each pass, can ensure that the appropriate amount of bone is taken (**Figure 7**).

Removal of acromial bone often aids viewing, particularly at the start of the resection, in patients with laterally sloping AC joints. In most patients, the clavicle can be clearly seen through the posterior viewing portal when resection is complete; however, the arthroscope can be moved to the anterior portal if necessary to directly visualize the joint and to ensure that no residual bone remains at the posterosuperior aspect of the clavicle. Periosteal soft tissue will be seen circumferentially surrounding the clavicular resection.

Direct Approach

The direct (superior) approach is less commonly used but may be appropriate in younger patients with distal clavicle osteolysis but no subacromial pathology. Technically, there is less working space available with the direct approach; therefore, a smaller diameter arthroscope and smaller instruments may be helpful.

Anterior and posterior portals into the AC joint are created, both for viewing and for resecting. With this approach, most of the joint capsule is left intact, which might allow earlier return to activities, but the important posterior ligaments are violated.

Débridement of soft tissue and bone is carried out, as with the inferior approach. Removal of soft tissue and meniscal remnants is important for adequate AC joint resection; however, an overly aggressive resection can lead to anteroposterior instability. The amount of bone resection recommended for distal clavicle excision has varied. Anatomic analysis indicates that the superior AC ligaments attach an average of 7.6 mm and 5.2 mm from the distal end of the clavicle in men and women, respectively.[2] Because these ligaments are most critical for anteroposterior stability of the clavicle,[3] excessive resection or soft-tissue release can increase anteroposterior motion and possibly cause distal clavicular pain. Arthroscopic resection should therefore be limited to approximately 5 mm to 7 mm of bone from the distal end of the clavicle. Resection of 5 mm of bone will effectively eliminate contact between the clavicle and acromion.[4] Removal of 1 mm to 3 mm of bone from the acromial facet will increase the effective resection of the clavicle without risking distal clavicle destabilization. It also can aid in visualization. Patients with a prior history of AC joint separation should be approached cautiously because underlying instability may be worsened by clavicular resection.

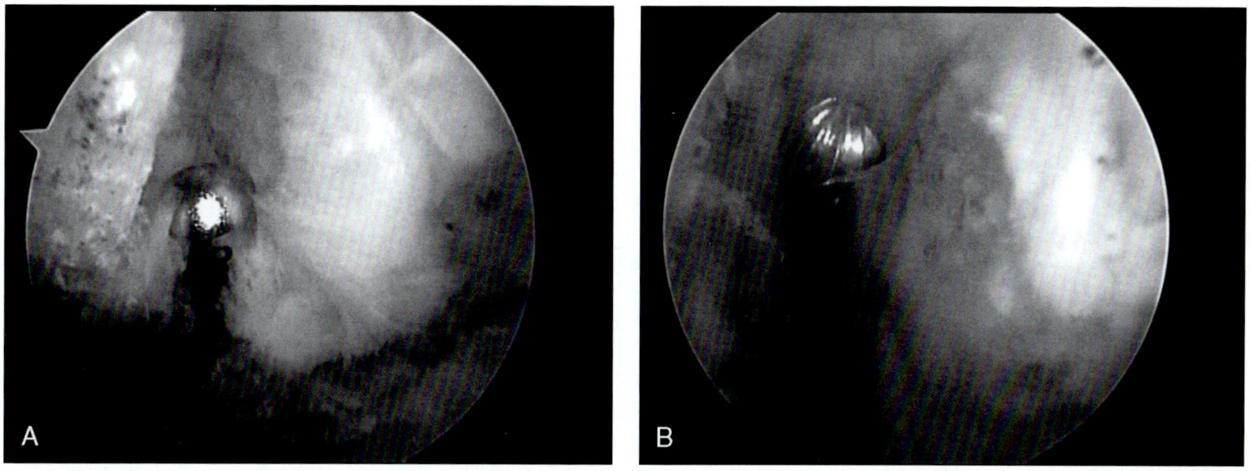

Figure 7 Arthroscopic images show soft-tissue resection at the distal clavicle, as viewed from the posterior portal.

Preventing Inadequate AC Joint Resection

Misdiagnosis can be prevented by careful review of the patient history, physical examination findings, and appropriate imaging studies. Inadequate resection can be prevented by good visualization and appropriate portal placement. Preoperative and postoperative radiographs of the AC joint should be taken to confirm adequate resection. Heterotopic ossification can occur after distal clavicle excision and might be confused with an inadequate resection if no postoperative radiographs are taken.[5] The surgeon should consider some type of prophylaxis in patients at risk for heterotopic ossification, such as those with spondylitic arthropathy.

Coplaning of the distal clavicle, which removes any inferior distal clavicle and medial acromial osteophytes and reduces any abrupt distal clavicle step-off, has been recommended by some authors for patients with impingement but no demonstrable AC joint pain.[6-8] Other authors, however, have suggested that disruption of the inferior capsule of the AC joint and partial resection of the AC joint capsule and meniscus can lead to AC joint pain in some patients.[6,9,10] This remains an area of controversy. Careful preoperative evaluation of the AC joint prior to acromioplasty is imperative. Coplaning without distal clavicle resection should be used with caution in patients who have a history of AC joint separation, significant degenerative changes, joint space narrowing, and cyst formation. AC joint disease may be a significant component of symptoms in these patients who have impingement syndrome, but diagnostic subacromial injection could relieve AC joint pain in a patient whose inferior acromioclavicular capsule has been disrupted by preexisting disease.

Case Management and Outcome Summary

The patient reported ongoing pain localized to the AC joint. Physical examination revealed pain at the AC joint with provocative maneuvers, but there were no other significant findings. Radiographs showed an inadequate AC joint resection, with posterosuperior bone visible at the distal clavicle. A diagnostic injection of 1% lidocaine into the AC joint completely relieved any residual pain.

The patient underwent revision arthroscopic AC joint resection 6 months after the initial surgery (**Figure 8**). A thorough intra-articular and subacromial evaluation was performed and revealed no other pathology. Postoperatively, the patient was able to return to all normal activities by 6 weeks, and by 4 months was pain free with all activities, including sports.

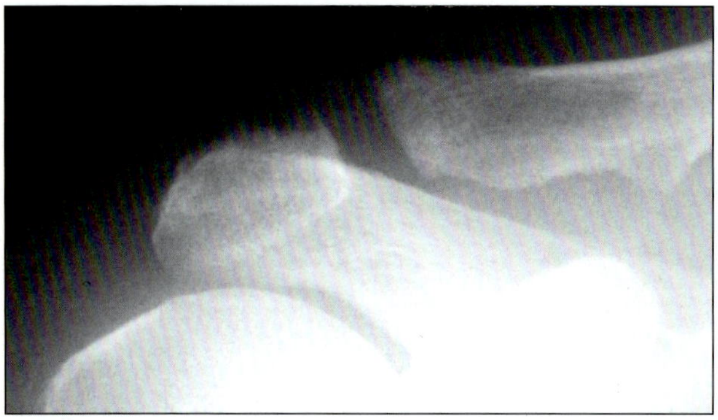

Figure 8 Revision of AC Joint resection.

STRATEGIES TO MINIMIZE COMMON COMPLICATIONS

Successful AC joint resection requires that the diagnosis be firmly established prior to surgery. The surgery is typically performed after failure of nonsurgical management consisting of activity modification, use of anti-inflammatory medications, and therapeutic lidocaine injections.

Arthroscopy should include a thorough intra-articular inspection to rule out other pathology as the source of shoulder pain. Resection of the AC joint can be performed through a direct or indirect approach, but good visualization of the distal clavicle is essential. Resection of the joint should include 2 mm to 3 mm of the acromial facet and approximately 5 mm of distal clavicle to ensure adequate resection without disruption of the AC ligaments. Patients with a known history of AC joint instability should be approached cautiously.

REFERENCES

1. Charron KM, Schepsis AA, Voloshin I: Arthroscopic distal clavicle resection in athletes: A prospective comparison of the direct and indirect approach. *Am J Sports Med* 2007;35:53-58.
2. Renfree KJ, Riley MK, Wheeler D, Hentz JG, Wright TW: Ligamentous anatomy of the distal clavicle. *J Shoulder Elbow Surg* 2003;12:355-359.
3. Klimkiewicz JJ, Williams GR, Sher JS, Karduna A, Des Jardins J, Iannotti JP: The acromioclavicular capsule as a restraint to posterior translation of the clavicle: A biomechanical analysis. *J Shoulder Elbow Surg* 1999;8:119-124.
4. Branch TP, Burdette HL, Shahriari AS, Carter FM, Hutton WC: The role of the acromioclavicular ligaments and the effect of distal clavicle resection. *Am J Sports Med* 1996;24:293-297.
5. Berg EE, Ciullo JV: Heterotopic ossification after acromioplasty and distal clavicle resection. *J Shoulder Elbow Surg* 1995;4:188-193.
6. Buford D Jr, Mologne T, McGrath S, Heinen G, Snyder S: Midterm results of arthroscopic co-planing of the acromioclavicular joint. *J Shoulder Elbow Surg* 2000;9:498-501.
7. Fischer BW, Gross RM, McCarthy JA, Arroyo JS: Incidence of acromioclavicular joint complications after arthroscopic subacromial decompression. *Arthroscopy* 1999;15:241-248.
8. Barber FA: Coplaning of the acromioclavicular joint. *Arthroscopy* 2001;17:913-917.
9. Barber FA: Long-term results of acromioclavicular joint coplaning. *Arthroscopy* 2006;22:125-129.
10. Rabalais RD, McCarty E: Surgical treatment of symptomatic acromioclavicular joint problems: A systematic review. *Clin Orthop Relat Res* 2007;455:30-37.

Chapter 7

Recurrent Instability After Arthroscopic Bankart Repair

Douglas H. Murray, MD

Case Presentation

A 24-year-old, right-handed man presented with recurrent shoulder instability following an anterior dislocation he sustained 2 years earlier during a motor vehicle accident. Radiographs of the shoulder showed a bony Bankart lesion. On physical examination, there was no evidence of generalized ligamentous laxity or multidirectional instability. The patient underwent closed reduction with intravenous sedation. An anterior-inferior labral tear with some bone involvement was noted on MRI scan (**Figure 1**). Nine months of rehabilitation, including dynamic shoulder stabilization, failed to alleviate the symptoms of instability.

Initial Surgery

An arthroscopic Bankart repair was performed, with placement of suture anchors on the anterior wall of the remaining glenoid rim. During the arthroscopy, the surgeon had difficulty determining exactly how much of the glenoid was missing. An attempt was made to pass the sutures around the bony tissue attached to the labrum.

Postoperatively, the patient progressed well initially and was pleased with his progress and lack of pain and instability. He continued to comply with the postoperative dynamic stabilization program and denied any specific repeat trauma to the shoulder.

Current Problem

Approximately 6 months after surgery, the patient developed a progressive sensation of apprehension with overhead activities. He described multiple subluxation episodes, which required self-manipulation reduction maneuvers on several occasions. Three weeks ago, he underwent a closed reduction after dislocating his shoulder while catching a football. He now reports good strength and function in any plane below the shoulder level, but notes pain and apprehension with any overhead activity.

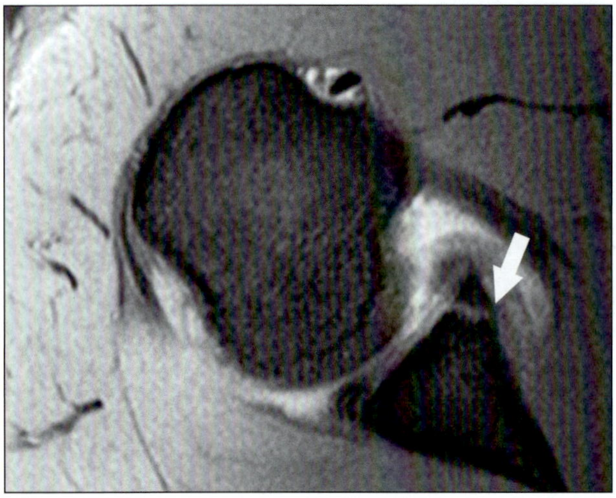

Figure 1 Axial MRI scan demonstrates a bony Bankart lesion (*arrow*).

Physical examination showed healed arthroscopic portal wounds, and there were no signs of inflammation, erythema, or atrophy of his shoulder girdle. He had no tenderness at the acromioclavicular joint and no bony prominences. The neck had full motion with no pain or radicular symptoms. Results of the distal neurovascular examination were negative, and deltoid function was normal. His rotator cuff strength was intact, and impingement signs were minimally positive.

Range-of-motion tests demonstrated forward elevation to 140°, limited by apprehension. He demonstrated external rotation in adduction to 50° and internal rotation to L3, both of which were equivalent to the contralateral left shoulder. An instability examination showed no ligamentous laxity at the elbow, wrist, or hand. The sulcus sign was trace positive bilaterally. The anterior apprehension test was markedly positive, with a positive relocation maneuver. The posterior apprehension test was negative. The anterior load and shift test showed grade 2+ instability, and the posterior load and shift test was trace positive.

Radiographs showed no evidence of arthritis or metallic suture anchors, but a Hill-Sachs deformity was noted. AP and axillary views demonstrated some anterior insufficiency of the glenoid rim, with anterior subluxation of the humeral head (**Figure 2**). An MRI scan demonstrated that there were no loose anchors; however, postsurgical changes at the anterior-inferior glenoid rim were noted, with a probable labral tear (**Figure 3**).

Bone insufficiency was suspected, but because this is difficult to evaluate definitively by MRI, a CT scan was obtained to evaluate the bone stock of the glenoid. The CT scan showed a defect of the anterior-inferior glenoid face involving approximately 35% of the articular surface (**Figure 4**). MRI revealed that the Hill-Sachs defect involved 20% of the circumference of the humeral head (**Figure 5**).

Discussion

The etiology of recurrent instability following arthroscopic Bankart repair is multifactorial.[1,2] Improved surgical techniques and appropriate patient selection have led to decreased recurrence rates for arthroscopic Bankart repair, which now match the 5% to 10% recurrence rates associated with open repair.[3-5] Recurrence rates are markedly lower for the patient who does not have significant bony defects or hyperlaxity of the ligaments; thus, this is the ideal patient for arthroscopic Bankart repair. Recurrence of instability can occur up to several years following the initial procedure.[1-5]

Recognizing Recurrent Instability

When a patient has recurrent instability after attempted surgical correction, the previous diagnosis, the surgical technique, and the postoperative regimen must be reevaluated to determine the possible etiologies (**Table 1**). Many patients who present with failed instability repair do so after another minor trauma; therefore, a thorough history and physical examination are important for determining whether this is indeed a new problem or a recurrence of the previous instability.

Ligamentous Laxity

In patients with failed instability repair, the degree of ligamentous laxity, the possibility of multidirectional instability, and the direction of unidirectional instability should be reassessed. The patient should also be reassessed for generalized ligamentous laxity. The

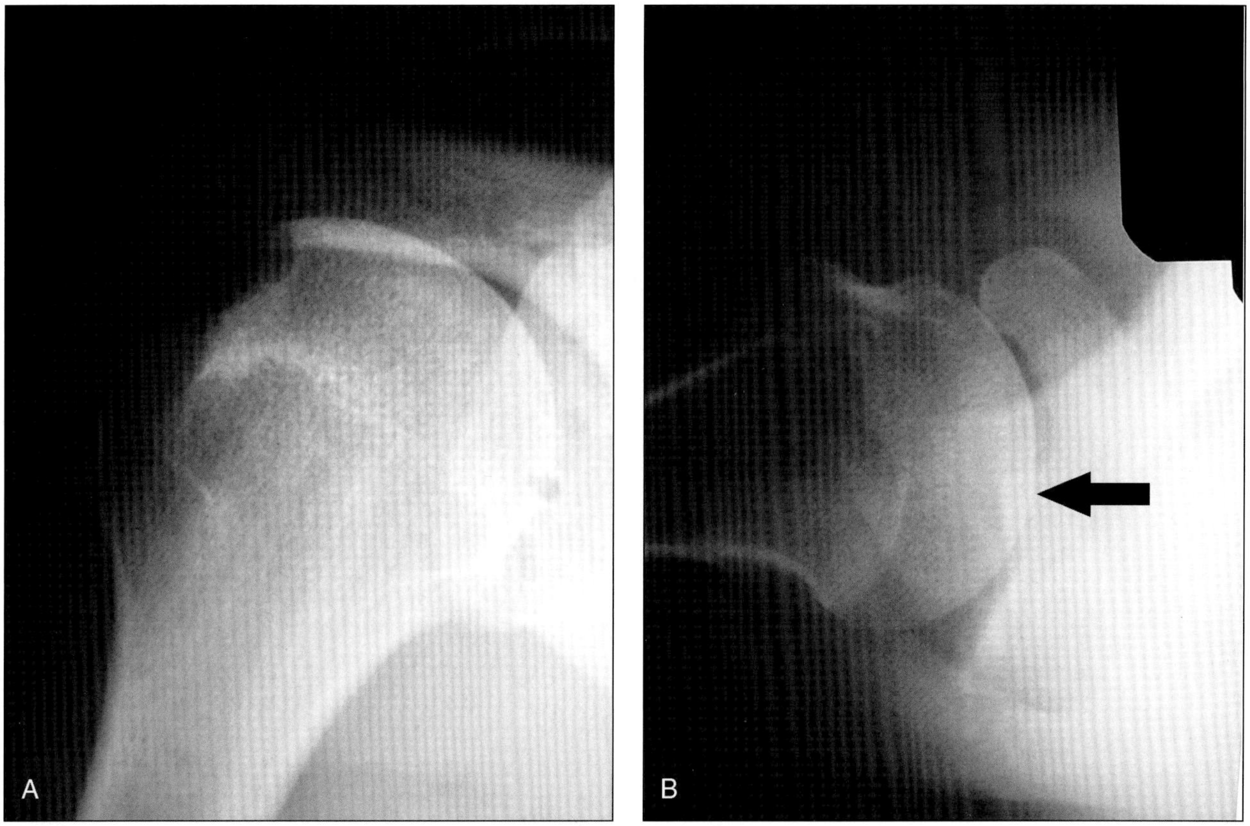

Figure 2 AP **(A)** and axillary **(B)** radiographs of the shoulder show anterior subluxation of the humeral head, with deficiency at the anterior glenoid rim. A Hill-Sachs deformity of the humeral head is also seen (*arrow*).

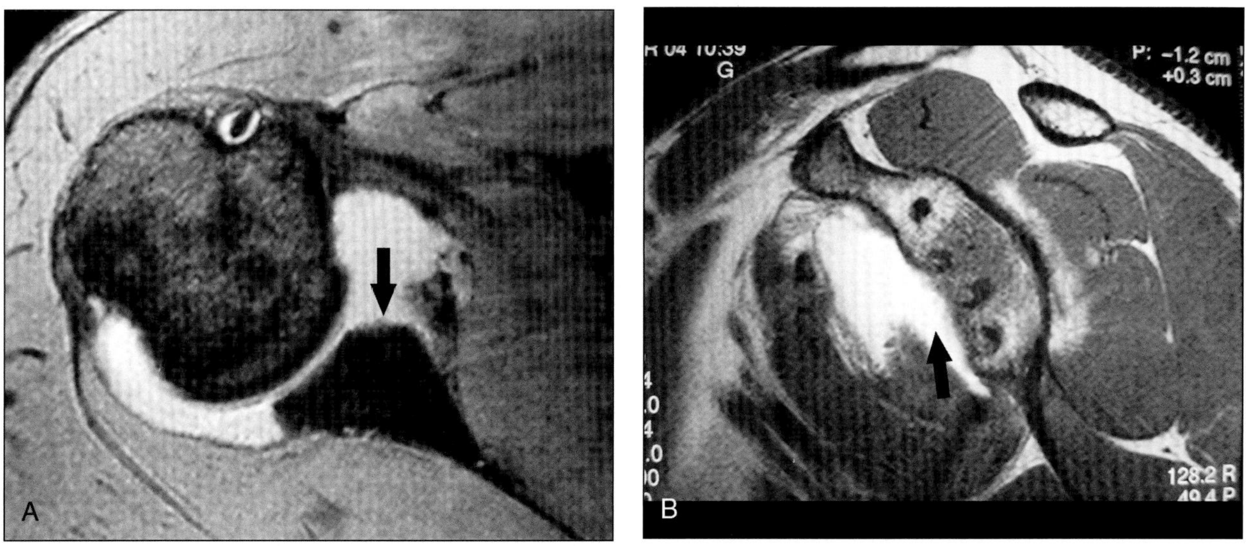

Figure 3 Axial **(A)** and sagittal **(B)** MRI scans reveal the bone defect at the glenoid (*arrows*).

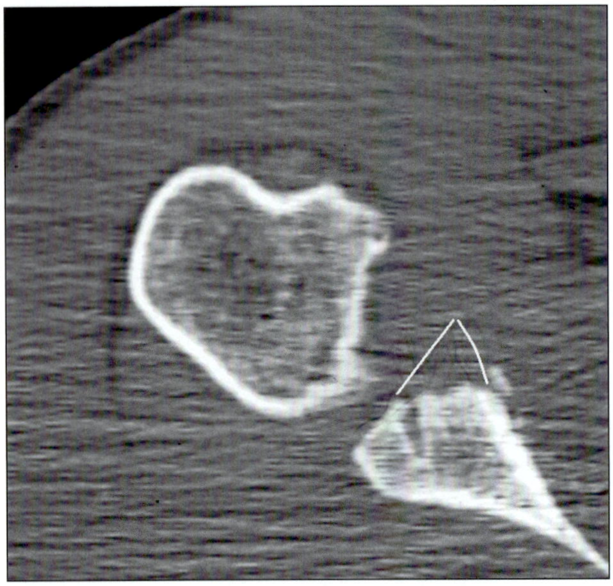

Figure 4 Axial CT scan confirms the bony deficiency at the glenoid.

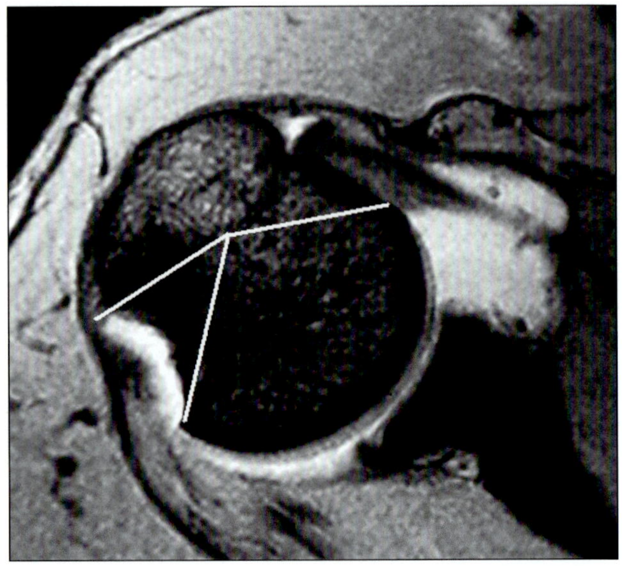

Figure 5 Axial MRI scan demonstrates a 20% circumferential defect on the humeral head.

Table 1: Differential Diagnosis for Failed Instability Repair

1. Misdiagnosis
- Anterior repair for multidirectional instability
- Anterior repair for posterior instability

2. Bone Deficiency
- Bankart lesion
- Engaging Hill-Sachs deformity

3. Capsulolabral Failure
- Loss of fixation
- Nonanatomic repair of labrum
- Capsular laxity not addressed
- Capsular deficiency
- Humeral capsular avulsion
- Intra-articular tear

4. Nerve palsy
- Axillary nerve

5. Ligamentous hyperlaxity syndrome
- Marfan syndrome
- Ehlers-Danlos syndrome

6. Habitual dislocator

anterior capsular tissues deform plastically before rupturing; therefore, some capsular laxity may be present even in patients with a Bankart lesion.[6] Careful evaluation of capsular laxity is important during Bankart repair to avoid incomplete correction of instability.

Collagen disorders, such as Ehlers-Danlos syndrome, put any instability repair at risk for failure because capsular tissues may stretch out again with time. Patients with diffuse capsular laxity will require imbrication of the capsule anteriorly, inferiorly, and posteriorly. Depending on patient preference and surgeon level of experience, however, this may be better treated with an open inferior capsular shift. In addition, an overtensioned unidirectional repair in a patient with multidirectional instability may lead to a fixed subluxation in the opposite direction and eventual failure of the instability repair.

Bone Deficiency

Significant glenoid bone deficiency, as seen in the case presentation, is a common cause of failure in arthroscopic Bankart repair.[1,2] Many acute bony Bankart lesions can be successfully addressed with arthroscopic stabilization, depending on bone fragment size and surgical technique.[7] This can be

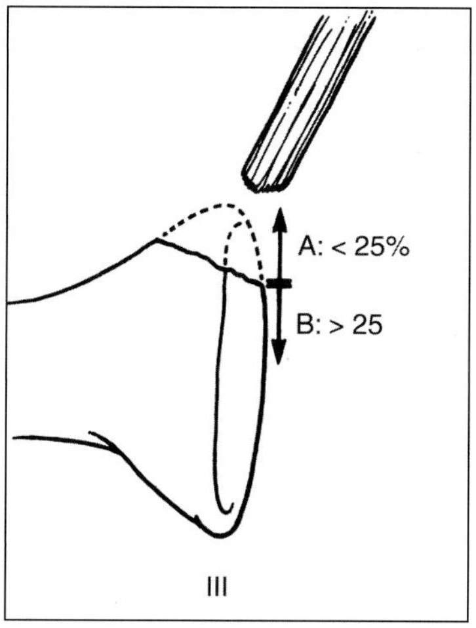

Figure 6 Bone defects involving less than 25% of the glenoid face may be addressed with a direct soft-tissue repair. (*Reproduced with permission from Bigliani LU, Newton PM, Steinmann SP, Connor PM, McIlveen SJ: Glenoid rim lesions associated with recurrent anterior dislocation of the shoulder.* Am J Sports Med *1998;26:41-45.*)

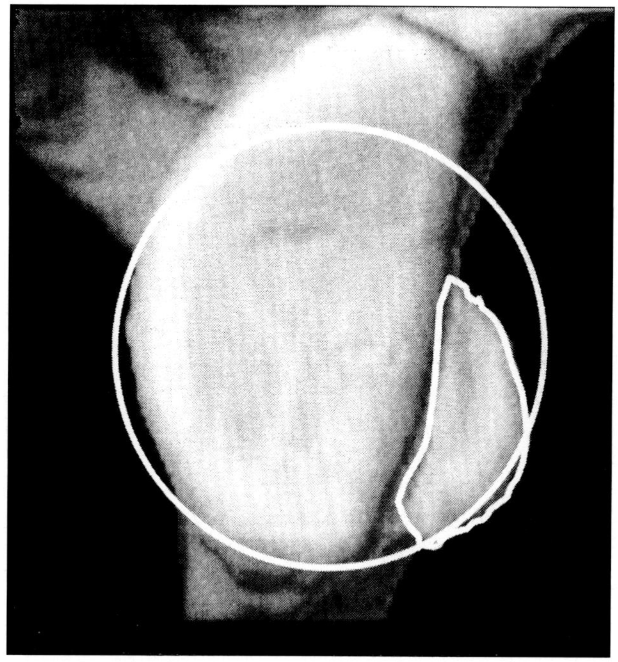

Figure 7 Three-dimensional CT reconstruction demonstrates the glenoid defect. (*Reproduced with permission from Sugaya H, Moriishi J, Dohi M, Kon Y, Tsuchiya A: Glenoid rim morphology in recurrent anterior glenohumeral instability.* J Bone Joint Surg Am *2003;85:878-884.*)

accomplished by incorporating the glenoid fragment into the anchor sutures and anatomically repositioning the bone onto the rim of the glenoid. Chronic glenoid defects can result from malunion of a glenoid rim fracture onto the anterior glenoid neck or from glenoid erosion caused by repetitive dislocation episodes. Most chronic glenoid defects are not of significant size, but careful evaluation is required, especially following failed instability repair. Typically, glenoid defects involving less than 25% of the articular surface can still be stabilized with a soft-tissue repair[8] (**Figure 6**). However, defects larger than this, or those that create an "inverted-pear" glenoid configuration, typically require open reconstruction.[2] Such defects are best assessed preoperatively on CT scans, particularly on three-dimensional reconstruction views with the humeral head subtracted out[9] (**Figure 7**). Intraoperative evaluation involves assessing the width of the glenoid relative to the central bare area and then comparing the anterior and posterior widths to calculate a relative deficiency measurement.[10] Arthroscopic assessment of the inverted-pear glenoid deformity is also possible.

Humeral head defects are typically not large enough to alter the surgical options in recurrent shoulder dislocations. Patients with chronically locked dislocations may have significant Hill-Sachs lesions that will change the surgical options. Defects involving more than 40% of the humeral head may require arthroplasty or osteoarticular allograft reconstruction.[11] Measurement of the defect is best performed on axial CT scans.[12] Despite recent interest and success in treating shoulder instability by reconstructing humeral head defects, most patients with instability can be managed effectively with adequate treatment of the capsulolabral and glenoid pathology.

Capsulolabral Failure

Capsulolabral insufficiency may be the result of an inadequate repair or a deficiency of capsulolabral tissue. Most anterior labral lesions involve the classic Bankart lesion; however, they may also include an intracapsular ligamentous tear or an avulsion of the capsule from the humeral insertion (humeral avulsion of the glenohumeral ligament [HAGL lesion]).[13-15] Capsular tissue deficiency may be encountered after multiple failed procedures, especially with failed thermal capsulorrhaphy. Wong and Williams[16] document-

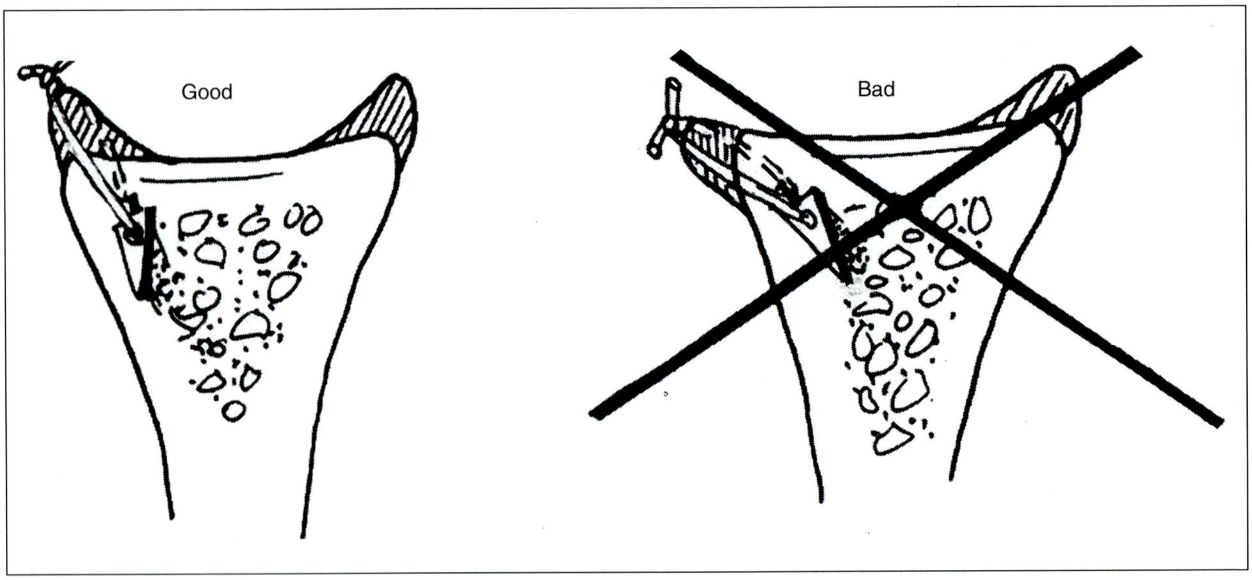

Figure 8 Anatomic placement of the labral repair requires placement of the suture anchors on the articular surface rather than on the anterior glenoid wall. (*Reproduced with permission from Boileau P, Villalba M, Héry JY, Balg F, Ahrens P, Neyton L: Risk factors for recurrence of shoulder instability after arthroscopic Bankart repair.* J Bone Joint Surg Am *2006;88:1755-1763.*)

ed attenuation of the capsular tissue in up to 20% of patients undergoing revision surgery for failed thermal instability repair. The presence of a HAGL lesion or capsular deficiency are indications for open instability repair because of the challenge of treating these lesions arthroscopically.

Voluntary Instability

Patients who voluntarily dislocate a shoulder for secondary gain may present with a failed surgical stabilization. This diagnosis must be ruled out before recommending any surgical intervention, especially revision repair. Typically, these patients will not respond to any surgical intervention—arthroscopic or open—and nonsurgical treatment and psychological evaluation are preferred.

Surgical Technique Errors

Even when the diagnosis and surgical plan are correct, surgical technique errors can lead to failure of arthroscopic Bankart repair. To achieve a successful result, the capsulolabral repair must involve anatomic fixation of the labrum to the glenoid rim and appropriate tensioning of the ligamentous structures. Repair of the Bankart lesion on the anterior glenoid neck rather than on the cartilaginous rim will lead to malpositioning of the labral tissue and a failure to recreate the anatomic concavity required for joint stability[17] (**Figure 8**). Placing buried suture anchors on the face of the anterior-inferior glenoid articular surface allows for recreation of the normal "bumper" of the anterior labrum, which augments the concavity of the glenoid surface. Provisional reduction of the labrum using a temporary suture or grasper allows the surgeon to plan anchor and suture placement. Appropriate lateral and superior advancement of the capsulolabral complex can be gauged by the tension of the anterior band of the inferior glenohumeral ligament. Elevation of the inferior capsule and labrum off the glenoid neck allows superior advancement and tensioning of the inferior capsule, even though suture anchors cannot be applied to the inferior glenoid rim.

Multiple suture anchors are typically necessary to achieve a stable Bankart repair. Boileau and associates[1] concluded that this factor was critical. Specifically, they found that patients with three or fewer anchors had higher rates of recurrent instability. Adequate fixation depends on appropriate anchor pullout strength, secure labral tissue capture, and appropriate suture loop and knot security. The purchase of each suture anchor should be tested after insertion by placing tension on the sutures manually.

Suture relay can be performed with a variety of devices, but the surgeon must confirm that the capsule and labrum held by the suture are of sufficient quality and quantity before tying the arthroscopic knots. The use of arthroscopic tacks has been abandoned because of complications associated with fracturing of the devices and foreign body reactions. The use of transglenoid sutures has also been abandoned because of complications with recurrence and trauma to the suprascapular nerve. Further tightening of the capsule and labral repair may be necessary in patients with hyperlaxity or significant plastic deformation of the capsule. Suture plication of the anterior capsule can be used to further tension the anterior capsule in these patients.

Rotator interval closure has also been promoted for additional tensioning of the capsule. The need for further tensioning can be evaluated intraoperatively by assessing the size of the inferior capsular pouch, a persistent drive-through sign, and by assessing the rotator interval size. The indication for these adjunctive maneuvers is not clearly defined, however, and overtensioning can occur. The risk of overtensioning can be minimized by placing the arm in 45° of external rotation during interval closure or capsular plication.

Nerve Palsy

Nerve palsy at the shoulder girdle can result in failure of the dynamic stabilization mechanism of the shoulder and recurrent instability. Preoperative assessment of deltoid and rotator cuff function is crucial because nerve injury can occur at the time of original injury or during surgical treatment. Using electrophysiological examination, nerve damage has been documented in 48% of anterior shoulder dislocations.[18]

If the patient's neurologic status is uncertain, a preoperative nerve conduction study of the shoulder should be performed. Nerve injury during surgery can occur with portal placement or during treatment of the capsule or labrum. Whereas cadaveric studies have clearly documented that the cephalic vein is at risk during shoulder arthroscopy procedures because of the vein's proximity to the anterior portals, there are conflicting reports on the proximity of important nerves to the shoulder portals. Some studies have reported that all nerves are safely more than 20 mm from all shoulder portals; however, other studies have documented that the axillary and musculocutaneous nerves are an average of 15 mm and 13 mm from the transsubscapularis 5 o'clock portal, respectively.[19-22]

If a thermal probe is used, the axillary nerve is at risk under the inferior capsule because the nerve is separated from the inferior capsule by an average of only 2.5 mm.[23] Rates of axillary neuropraxia between 1.4% and 21% after thermal capsulorrhaphy have been reported.[24,25] Risk of axillary nerve injury with suture passage must be considered, but has not been reported. Suprascapular nerve injury has been reported with the use of transglenoid sutures. This nerve is also at risk with dissection around the spinoglenoid notch if a perilabral cyst is decompressed arthroscopically. With updated techniques, it appears that the risk of nerve injury from portal placement can be minimized by avoiding the 5 o'clock portal and avoiding overuse of the thermal probe on the capsule.

Inadequate or Inappropriate Rehabilitation

Finally, the patient's postoperative rehabilitation program must be evaluated to rule this out as a cause for treatment failure. The damaged capsular tissues require proprioceptive reeducation, and the dynamic stabilizers of the shoulder joint must be reconditioned as well. Secure, anatomic fixation has been shown to allow immediate rehabilitation and motion without adverse effect.[26]

With appropriate rehabilitation, range of motion is generally increased as tolerated while the at-risk position of abduction external rotation is avoided for 3 months. Excessive tension on the healing labrum must be avoided until adequate soft-tissue-to-bone healing has occurred. Gentle rotator cuff and periscapular strengthening as well as proprioceptive exercises are allowed approximately 6 weeks after surgery. Contact sports should generally be avoided for 6 months.

Managing Recurrent Stability

Nonsurgical treatment might be an option for patients with recurrent instability after arthroscopic

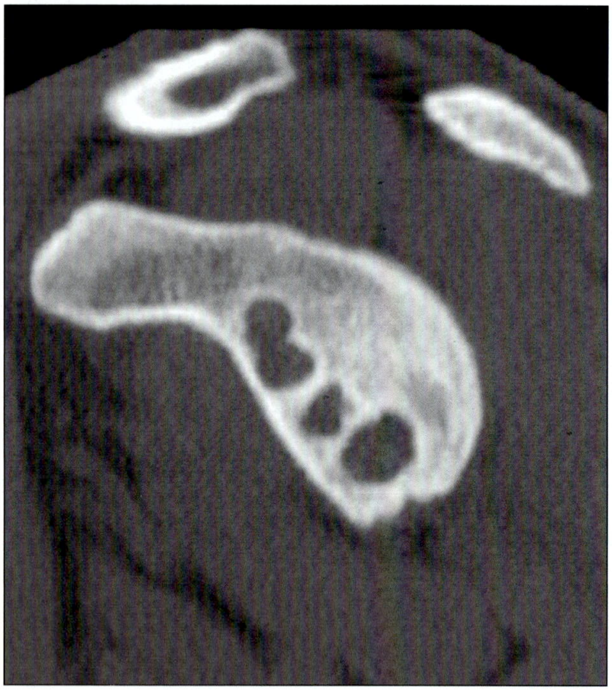

Figure 9 Coalescence of osteolytic lesions around absorbable suture anchors can lead to subacute anchor loosening. (*Reproduced with permission from Athwal GS, Shridharani SM, O'Driscoll SW: Osteolysis and arthropathy of the shoulder after use of bioabsorbable knotless suture anchors: A report of four cases.* J Bone Joint Surg Am *2006;88:1840-1845.*)

Bankart repair if the rehabilitation program was incomplete. However, if an appropriate dynamic stabilization and proprioceptive program do not alleviate symptoms, then revision surgery may be necessary.

After assessing for the problems discussed previously, each potential source of recurrence must be addressed during surgical revision. Arthroscopic revision can be successful if the specific causes of recurrent instability can be addressed adequately.[27] Arthroscopic revision can be considered if adequate bone and capsulolabral structures are present. If the bone defect is significant, or if a soft-tissue deficit such as a HAGL lesion or capsular deficiency is diagnosed, open reconstruction may be required.

Recurrence of a true Bankart soft-tissue lesion can be revised arthroscopically if other sources of recurrent instability have been ruled out. Repeat trauma on a healed labral repair can occur; however, the history and physical examination must carefully rule out other sources of recurrence. Revision labral repair is facilitated if bioabsorbable anchors have resorbed without an osteolytic lesion. Coalescence of osteolytic lesions around absorbable anchors can lead to late loosening of the anchor and can complicate placement of revision anchors[28] (**Figure 9**). Implanted metallic suture anchors will have to be avoided for the revision procedure.

Significant bone deficiency, as seen in the case presentation, must be addressed through an open reconstruction. The concavity-compression mechanism of shoulder stability depends on both the soft-tissue restraints and the bony architecture of the shoulder. Soft-tissue reconstruction alone in a patient with significant glenoid defects will fail because there is no compensation for the loss of bony concavity. Options for patients with a glenoid defect include a coracoid transfer with revision capsular repair.[2,29] Other bone-graft options for the glenoid defect include autogenous or allograft iliac crest bone, with contouring of the cortical bone to help restore the appropriate concavity.[30] Preoperative measurement of the width of the glenoid vault by CT scan can help predict the accurate length of the cannulated screws needed to fix the graft to the anterior glenoid rim.

Hill-Sachs defects rarely require specific intervention; however, engaging humeral head defects can be addressed by tuberosity transfer, osteoarticular allograft, or arthroplasty if the defect is large enough (approximately > 40% of the articular surface).[11,31]

Capsular tissue deficiency can lead to failure of revision stabilization. Allograft tissue should be available if the patient has a history of multiple failed procedures or a failed thermal capsulorrhaphy[32,33] (**Figure 10**). An Achilles tendon graft with a bone block can be used to simultaneously reconstruct a glenoid defect and deficient anterior capsular tissues.

Case Management and Outcome Summary

The patient had a failed arthroscopic instability repair as a result of bony insufficiency at the anterior-inferior glenoid articular surface. There was a loss of concavity compression, which cannot be compensated for by a soft-tissue procedure alone. The patient underwent a coracoid transfer and revision capsulorrhaphy.

Three suture anchors were placed on the existing glenoid rim at the articular surface, and the coracoid transfer was secured with two cannulated, partially threaded screws (**Figure 11**). The capsular repair includes repairing the anterior-inferior labrum with a capsular shift if needed. The coracoid transfer is placed extra-articularly relative to the capsular repair.

Postoperatively the patient was immobilized for 2 weeks, after which active-assisted forward elevation to 90° and neutral external rotation were allowed. At 6 weeks postoperatively, he was allowed to increase forward elevation as tolerated with the arm internally rotated. External rotation in adduction was increased to tolerance as well. Abduction with external rotation was not allowed until 3 months postoperatively.

By 3 months, the patient regained 165° of forward elevation and 40° of external rotation with the arm at the side. By 5 months postoperatively, he was comfortable with overhead activities and had no symptoms of instability.

Strategies to Minimize Complications

Recurrence of instability after arthroscopic Bankart repair can result from a variety of factors; therefore, simply repeating the same procedure will not typically resolve the problem. All possible etiologies must be considered, and the patient's anatomic and functional deficiencies must be resolved.

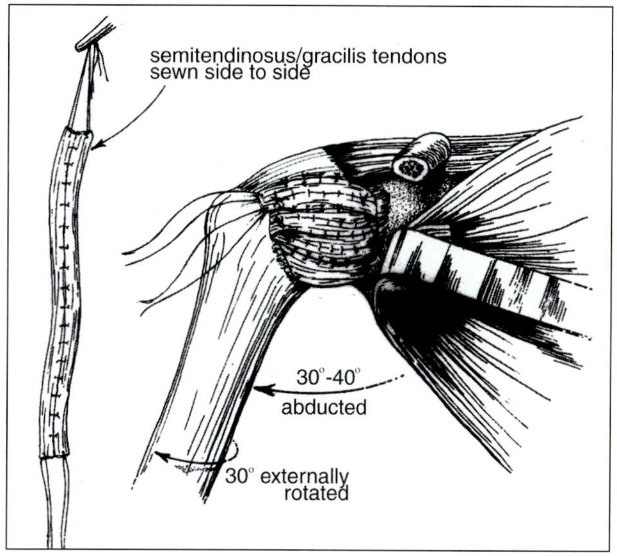

Figure 10 Allograft reconstruction of deficient capsular tissue. (*Reproduced with permission from Warner JPJ, Venegas AA, Lehtinen JT, Macy JJ: Management of capsular deficiency of the shoulder.* J Bone Joint Surg Am *2002;85:1668-1671.*)

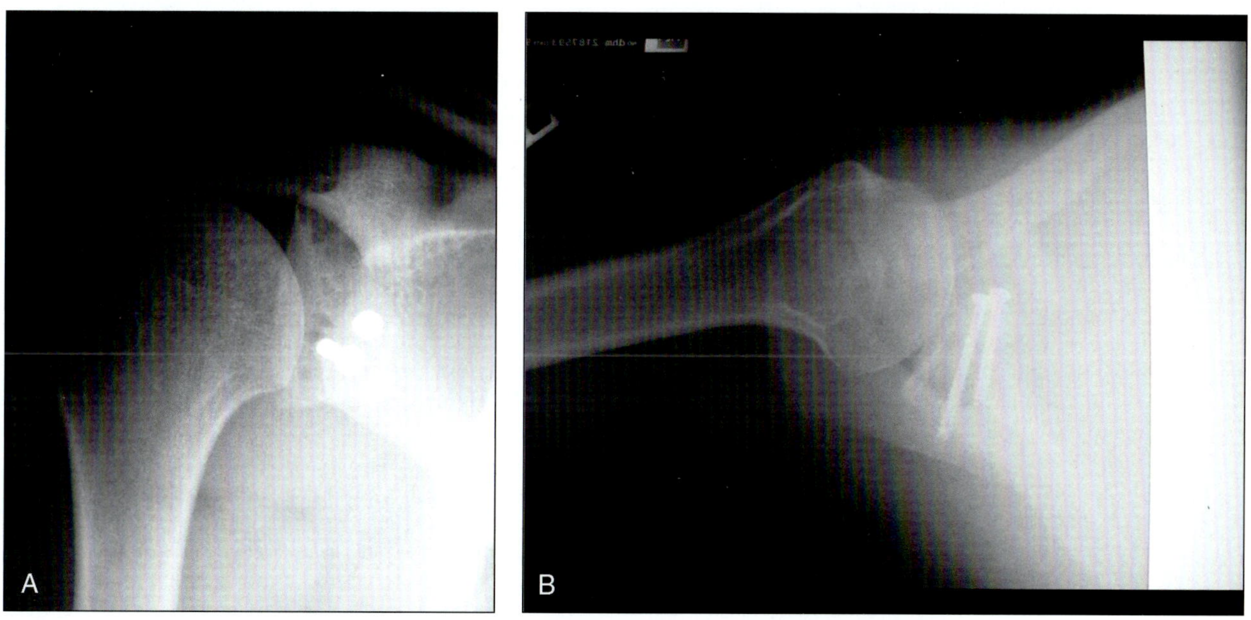

Figure 11 AP **(A)** and axillary **(B)** radiographs following coracoid transfer and capsulorrhaphy.

Evaluation of failed instability repair includes a careful history and physical examination in addition to appropriate imaging studies to determine the source of recurrence. Preoperative assessment of the index procedure must include the evaluation of bone defects, capsulolabral structures, and current neurovascular status to prevent failure. Arthroscopic revision may suffice after failure of an arthroscopic instability repair; however, open reconstruction may be required for patients with significant bony or capsular deficiency.

References

1. Boileau P, Villalba M, Héry JY, Balg F, Ahrens P, Neyton L: Risk factors for recurrence of shoulder instability after arthroscopic Bankart repair. *J Bone Joint Surg Am* 2006;88:1755-1763.
2. Burkhart SS, De Beer JF: Traumatic glenohumeral bone defects and their relationship to failure of arthroscopic Bankart repairs: Significance of the inverted-pear glenoid and the humeral engaging Hill-Sachs lesion. *Arthroscopy* 2000;16:677-694.
3. Fabbriciani C, Milano G, Demontis A, Fadda S, Ziranu F, Mulas PD: Arthroscopic versus open treatment of Bankart lesion of the shoulder: A prospective randomized study. *Arthroscopy* 2004;20:456-462.
4. Gartsman GM, Roddey TS, Hammerman SM: Arthroscopic treatment of anterior-inferior instability: Two to five-year follow-up. *J Bone Joint Surg Am* 2000;82:991-1003.
5. Kim SH, Ha KI, Cho YB, Ryu BD, Oh I: Arthroscopic anterior stabilization of the shoulder: Two to six-year follow-up. *J Bone Joint Surg Am* 2003;85:1511-1518.
6. Bigliani LU, Pollock RG, Soslowsky LJ, Flatow EL, Pawluk RJ, Mow VC: Tensile properties of the glenohumeral ligament. *J Orthop Res* 1992;10:187-197.
7. Sugaya H, Moriishi J, Kanisawa I, Tsuchiya A: Arthroscopic osseous Bankart repair for chronic recurrent traumatic anterior glenohumeral instability. *J Bone Joint Surg Am* 2005;87:1752-1760.
8. Bigliani LU, Newton PM, Steinmann SP, Connor PM, McIlveen SJ: Glenoid rim lesions associated with recurrent anterior dislocation of the shoulder. *Am J Sports Med* 1998;26:41-45.
9. Sugaya H, Moriishi J, Dohi M, Kon Y, Tsuchiya A: Glenoid rim morphology in recurrent anterior glenohumeral instability. *J Bone Joint Surg Am* 2003;85:878-884.
10. Burkhart SS, DeBeer JF, Tehrany AM, Parten PM: Quantifying glenoid bone loss arthroscopically in shoulder instability. *Arthroscopy* 2002;18:488-491.
11. Gerber C, Lambert SM: Allograft reconstruction of segmental defects of the humeral head for the treatment of chronic locked posterior dislocation of the shoulder. *J Bone Joint Surg Am* 1996;78:376-382.
12. Cicak N: Posterior dislocation of the shoulder. *J Bone Joint Surg Br* 2004;86:324-332.
13. Bokor DJ, Conboy VB, Olson C: Anterior instability of the glenohumeral joint with humeral avulsion of the glenohumeral ligament: A review of 41 cases. *J Bone Joint Surg Br* 1999;81:93-96.
14. Mizuno N, Yoneda M, Hayashida K, Nakagawa S, Mae T, Izawa K: Recurrent anterior shoulder dislocation caused by a midsubstance complete capsular tear. *J Bone Joint Surg Am* 2005;87:2717-2723.
15. Rhee YG, Ha JH, Park KJ: Clinical outcome of anterior shoulder instability with capsular midsubstance tear: A comparison of isolated midsubstance tear and midsubstance tear with Bankart lesion. *J Shoulder Elbow Surg* 2006;15:586-590.
16. Wong KL, Williams GR: Complications of thermal capsulorrhaphy of the shoulder. *J Bone Joint Surg Am* 2001;83:151-155.
17. Harryman DT, Ballmer FP, Harris SL, Sidles JA: Arthroscopic labral repair to the glenoid rim. *Arthroscopy* 1994;10:20-30.
18. Visser CP, Coene LN, Brand R, Tavy DL: The incidence of nerve injury in anterior dislocation of the shoulder and its influence on functional recovery: A prospective clinical and EMG study. *J Bone Joint Surg Br* 1999;81:679-685.
19. Davidson PA, Tibone JE: Anterior-inferior (5 o'clock) portal for shoulder arthroscopy. *Arthroscopy* 1995;11:519-525.
20. Lo IK, Lind CC, Burkhart SS: Glenohumeral arthroscopy portals established using an outside-in technique: Neurovascular anatomy at risk. *Arthroscopy* 2004;20:596-602.
21. Meyer M, Graveleau N, Hardy P, Landreau P: Anatomic risks of shoulder arthroscopy portals: Anatomic cadaveric study of 12 portals. *Arthroscopy* 2007;23:529-536.
22. Gelber PE, Reina F, Caceres E, Monllau JC: A comparison of risk between the lateral decubitus and the beach-chair position when establishing an anteroinferior shoulder portal: A cadaveric study. *Arthroscopy* 2007;23:522-528.
23. Price MR, Tillett ED, Acland RD, Nettleton GS: Determining the relationship of the axillary nerve to the shoulder joint capsule from an arthroscopic perspective. *J Bone Joint Surg Am* 2004;86:2135-2142.

24. Wong KL, Williams GR: Complications of thermal capsulorrhaphy of the shoulder. *J Bone Joint Surg Am* 2001;83(suppl 2):151-155.
25. Miniaci A, McBirnie J: Thermal capsular shrinkage for treatment of multidirectional instability of the shoulder. *J Bone Joint Surg Am* 2003;85:2283-2287.
26. Kim SH, Ha KI, Jung MW, Lim MS, Kim YM, Park JH: Accelerated rehabilitation after arthroscopic Bankart repair for selected cases: A prospective randomized clinical study. *Arthroscopy* 2003;19:722-731.
27. Kim SH, Ha SI, Kim YM: Arthroscopic revision Bankart repair: A prospective outcome study. *Arthroscopy* 2002;18:469-482.
28. Athwal GS, Shridharani SM, O'Driscoll SW: Osteolysis and arthropathy of the shoulder after use of bioabsorbable knotless suture anchors: A report of four cases. *J Bone Joint Surg Am* 2006;88:1840-1845.
29. Allain J, Goutallier D, Glorion C: Long-term results of the Latarjet procedure for the treatment of anterior instability of the shoulder. *J Bone Joint Surg Am* 1998;80:841-852.
30. Millett PJ, Clavert P, Warner JJP: Open operative treatment for anterior shoulder instability: When and why? *J Bone Joint Surg Am* 2005;87:419-432.
31. Yagishita K, Thomas BJ: Use of allograft for large Hill-Sachs lesion associated with anterior glenohumeral dislocation. *Injury* 2002;33:791-794.
32. Iannotti JP, Antoniou J, Williams GR, Ramsey ML: Iliotibial band reconstruction for treatment of glenohumeral instability associated with irreparable capsular deficiency. *J Shoulder Elbow Surg* 2002;11:618-623.
33. Warner JPJ, Venegas AA, Lehtinen JT, Macy JJ: Management of capsular deficiency of the shoulder. *J Bone Joint Surg Am* 2002;85:1668-1671.

Chapter 8

Failed Arthroscopic SLAP Repair

Douglas H. Murray, MD

Case Presentation

A 21-year-old, right-handed female volleyball player presented with right posterior shoulder pain and weakness with overhead activities, specifically in the late cocking phase of movement. Physical examination demonstrated normal neurologic function, and her shoulder exhibited no visible asymmetry, atrophy, or tenderness to palpation. Shoulder motion was normal, but she had pain at full elevation. Rotator cuff strength was intact. Pain was maximized during the compression-rotation test and the anterior apprehension test but was relieved with a relocation maneuver. Both shoulders demonstrated a grade 1 sulcus sign, with 1 cm of translation. Routine radiographs of the affected shoulder were normal, but an MR arthrogram demonstrated a possible superior labrum anterior to posterior (SLAP) tear without signs of a rotator cuff tear or perilabral cyst (**Figure 1**).

Initial treatment consisted of 6 weeks of rest, followed by a supervised dynamic shoulder stabilization program and posterior capsular stretching. After 6 months of treatment, during which time she had persistent pain and was unable to participate in athletic activity, she elected to proceed with diagnostic arthroscopy and arthroscopic SLAP repair.

Initial Surgery

Examination under anesthesia demonstrated a 1-cm sulcus sign, but otherwise no dramatic instability. Diagnostic arthroscopy documented a greater than 5-mm separation of the anterior and posterior aspects of the superior labrum off the glenoid rim. The proximal biceps tendon was benign, and there was no rotator cuff pathology. The capsulolabral complex showed a normal attachment anteriorly and inferiorly, but a drive-through sign was noted (**Figure 2**). There was no abnormality of the rotator interval.

A SLAP repair was performed after the superior glenoid rim was débrided down to bleeding bone using a full-radius resector in the anterosuperior portal. An anteroinferior portal was created for suture management. The labrum was repaired with one suture anchor seated anterior to the biceps

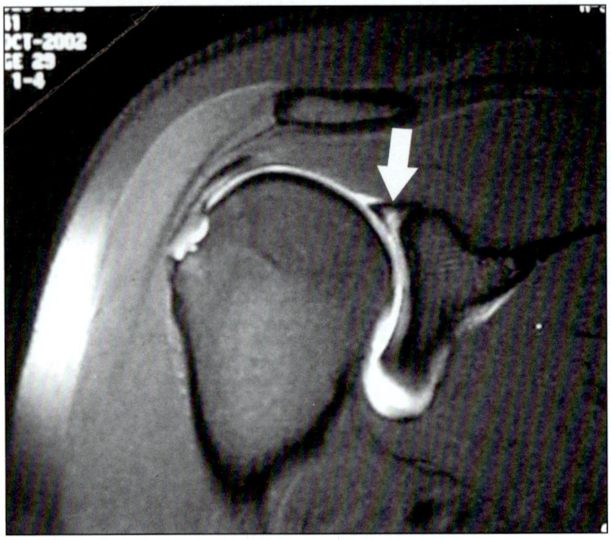

Figure 1 MRI scan demonstrates a superior labral tear.

origin on the prepared glenoid rim (**Figure 3**). Suture relay was completed through the anterior labral base of the biceps origin by passing the relay device through the anterosuperior portal and retrieving it from the anteroinferior portal. A sliding locking knot was used to secure the labrum to the superior glenoid such that at the end of the procedure the labrum was directly apposed to the glenoid rim. The drive-through sign was improved but still mildly present.

The patient was immobilized in a sling for 2 weeks, after which physical therapy was initiated. For the first 4 weeks, she was allowed forward elevation to 90° and external rotation to neutral with the arm adducted. At 6 weeks postoperatively, she was allowed to increase elevation and external rotation as tolerated; however, the abducted externally rotated position was avoided.

Despite compliance with the physical therapy regimen, the patient was unable to regain full forward elevation and noted persistent pain in the posterior shoulder region with increasing use of the arm. Examination showed full active-assisted motion, but she had significant pain with any resistance to forward elevation above the shoulder level and marked posterior shoulder pain with the anterior apprehension test that improved with the relocation maneuver. There were no overt signs of infection.

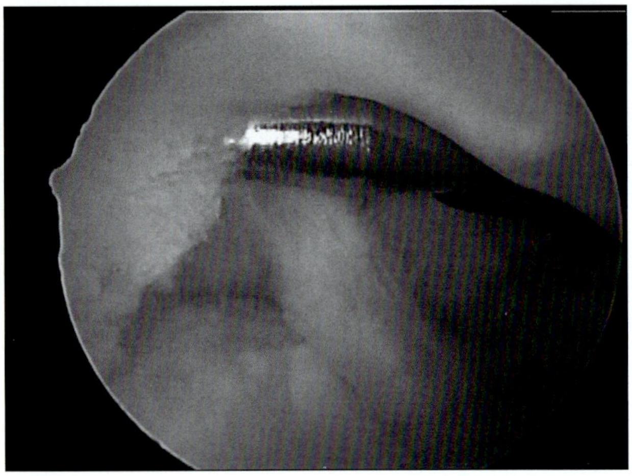

Figure 2 Arthroscopic examination confirms a type II SLAP lesion.

Current Problem and Treatment

After 6 months with persistent pain and incomplete recuperation of strength and motion, a repeat MR arthrogram was obtained. The suture anchor appeared stable, but the superior labrum showed postsurgical changes with persistence of the SLAP lesion from 10 o'clock to 1 o'clock. The labrum was not healed at the site of repair, and there appeared to be more involvement posterior to the biceps origin (**Figure 4**). The diagnosis was a symptomatic, persistent SLAP lesion status post attempted repair. The patient elected to proceed with diagnostic arthroscopy and revision repair.

Discussion

Lesions of the superior labrum have been recognized as an isolated or concomitant source of shoulder pathology.[1-3] SLAP lesions may be caused by acute injury or by repetitive trauma from overhead activities.

Surgical repair of isolated type II SLAP lesions has been shown to predictably alleviate related symptoms in 76% to 91% of patients.[4,5] Débridement without repair of a SLAP lesion may provide temporary relief for patients who engage in overhead activities, but the results deteriorate significantly within 3 years.[6] It can be difficult to interpret the results for SLAP repairs because patients frequently have con-

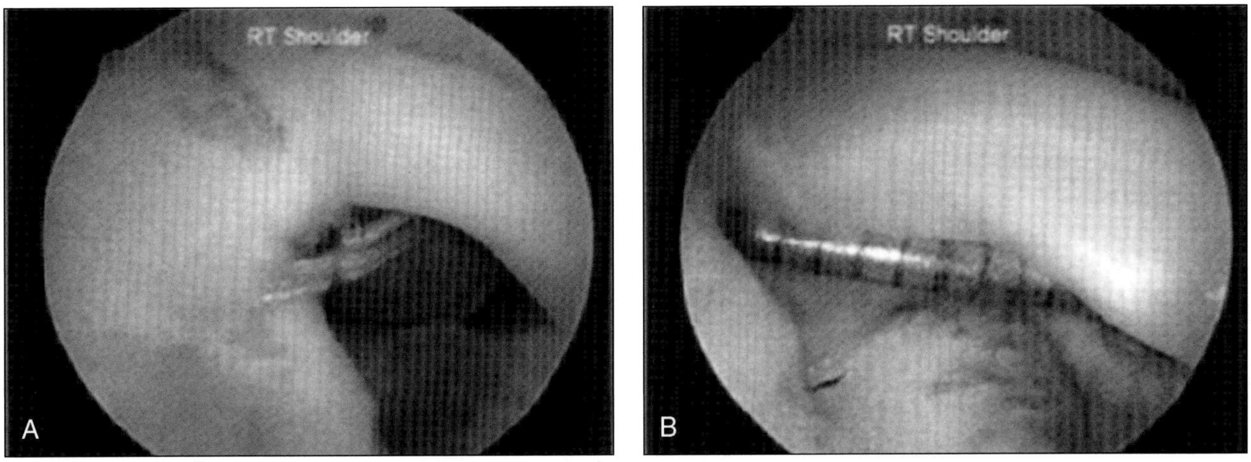

Figure 3 A suture anchor is placed at the anterior margin of the biceps origin **(A)** and tied to secure the labrum to the glenoid rim **(B)**.

comitant shoulder pathology, such as instability or rotator cuff tearing.

Diagnosing SLAP Lesions

SLAP lesions can be challenging to diagnose because patients may have overlapping shoulder pathology and because the results of the physical examination and other diagnostic studies may be difficult to interpret. Definitive diagnosis of a SLAP tear can be made only with arthroscopic examination of the shoulder.

Clinical Features

SLAP lesions have been classified by Snyder,[2] with a subclassification of type II lesions by Burkhart and Morgan.[7] In many patients, there is no one specific finding on physical or radiographic examination that can reliably be used to make the diagnosis of a SLAP tear. Clinical diagnosis is based on the patient history, several physical examination findings, and MR imaging. Each of these factors can vary with individual patients.

In the nonathlete, SLAP tears are typically caused by a fall on an outstretched hand or by a distraction mechanism with the shoulder in abduction and external rotation. Athletes, such as baseball pitchers, who engage in repetitive overhead throwing can present with a sudden onset of pain, or a gradual onset of pain may be noted. In athletes, the symptoms of a

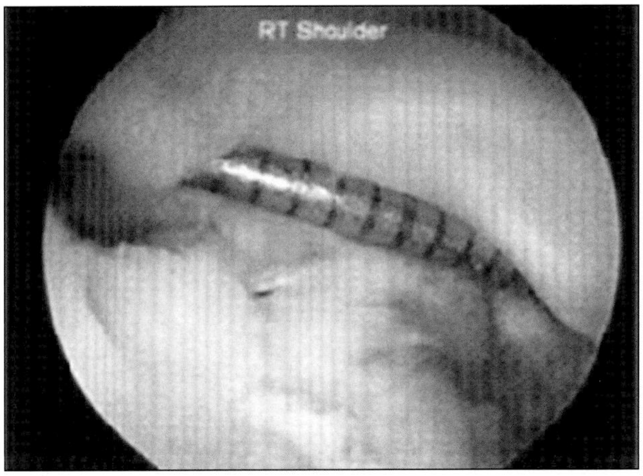

Figure 4 Example of a persistent SLAP lesion posterior to the biceps origin, despite repair of the anterior portion of the SLAP lesion.

SLAP lesion include pain with overhead activities, loss of strength or velocity, or painful clicking in the shoulder.[5,8]

The most common clinical finding in patients with a SLAP lesion is a positive compression-rotation test.[5,9] Other frequently associated findings include posterior shoulder pain with the anterior apprehension test that is relieved by the relocation test[10] and a positive biceps load test.[11] Unfortunately, there is no single perfect test for diagnosing SLAP lesions. In a study of 426 patients who underwent shoulder arthroscopy, McFarland and associates[12] found that the incidence of positive preoperative examination results was not statistically different between patients with or without SLAP lesions. In an electromyographic analysis of the biceps during SLAP examination maneuvers, Swaringen and associates[13] demonstrated that the signal at the long head of the biceps was maximized during the active-compression test and during the biceps tension test (Speed test); therefore, these tests may be the best for isolating pathology at the biceps long head tendon.

The accuracy of MR evaluation of SLAP lesions has been reported to be as high as 98% sensitivity and specificity; however, a report by nonorthopaedic community radiologists[14] documented rates of 50% sensitivity and 69% specificity, demonstrating the potential difficulties in interpreting MRI studies.

Because patients with SLAP lesions can have any number of positive findings among the tests mentioned, diagnosis should be based on a review of the entire clinical scenario. Typically, the mechanism of injury (acute or chronic) raises the suspicion for a SLAP lesion, and a number of characteristic findings on physical examination and other studies help to substantiate the diagnosis. The definitive diagnosis of a SLAP lesion and its classification is not made until diagnostic arthroscopy.

Recognizing a Failed SLAP Repair

Failed SLAP repairs can be even more challenging to evaluate. Diagnostic studies that are not perfect preoperatively may be even less predictable after surgery because of postsurgical changes. The original diagnosis, surgical technique, and rehabilitation compliance must all be assessed. Concomitant pathology needs to be ruled out because acromioclavicular pathology, glenohumeral instability, perilabral cysts, and rotator cuff tears can mimic the symptoms of a SLAP lesion.

Even with the correct diagnosis, failure of the SLAP repair can occur as a result of many factors, including inadequate initial fixation, loss of adequate fixation, or inappropriate rehabilitation. Inadequate initial fixation can be attributed to insecure suture anchor placement, lack of secure fixation as a result of suturing technique, or an inadequate number of fixation points of the lesion. However, even with adequate fixation, a SLAP repair may still fail if the glenoid rim is not properly prepared to allow labral healing, if a suture anchor is located incorrectly or loosens during rehabilitation, or if suture knot security fails.

Rehabilitation following SLAP repair focuses on preventing stiffness while avoiding strain on the repair. Abduction with external rotation is typically avoided for the first 12 weeks; the other planes of motion are gradually increased. Shoulder strengthening is achieved through isometrics, scapular stabilization, and a rotator cuff program.

Persistent pain following SLAP repair should be evaluated with a thorough history and physical examination. MR arthrogram is the study of choice to assess the labrum and other structures, although postsurgical changes will decrease the accuracy of interpreting a persistent or recurrent SLAP lesion.

Managing the Failed SLAP Repair

Once the diagnosis of a failed SLAP repair has been confirmed arthroscopically, revision repair of the lesion is the most predictable treatment for the overhead athlete. Other options include labral débridement, biceps tenodesis, or biceps tenotomy. These options may suffice in the patient who doesn't participate in overhead activities; however, they are not ideal for restoring the shoulder biomechanics needed by the young athlete. In this patient population, the "peel back" of the posterior labrum associated with the SLAP lesion needs to be corrected to restore normal shoulder mechanics for overhead throwing.

Surgical Technique

It is not feasible to place the posterior suture anchor via the anterior portal; rather, this is best accomplished through the portal of Wilmington (accessory lateral portal).[7] This portal is developed by making an incision approximately 1 cm lateral and 1 cm anterior to the posterolateral corner of the acromion. The angle is confirmed by a percutaneous spinal needle, typically aimed toward the middle of the coracoid. Percutaneous insertion of the posterior suture anchor without a cannula is recommended to minimize trauma to the rotator cuff muscle-tendon junction, which must be perforated.[15] Suture relay is per-

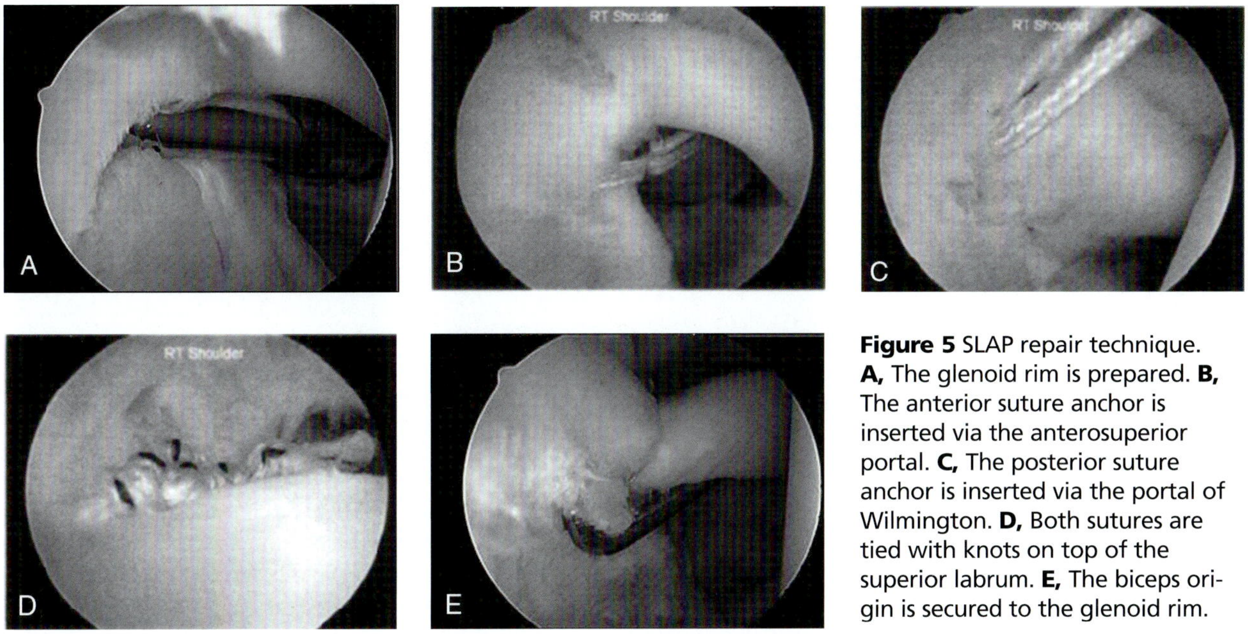

Figure 5 SLAP repair technique. **A,** The glenoid rim is prepared. **B,** The anterior suture anchor is inserted via the anterosuperior portal. **C,** The posterior suture anchor is inserted via the portal of Wilmington. **D,** Both sutures are tied with knots on top of the superior labrum. **E,** The biceps origin is secured to the glenoid rim.

formed with penetrating suture graspers or with a suture relay device from the anterior or accessory lateral portal. A second anterior portal is typically required for suture management. Anterior anchors may be inserted accurately from the anterosuperior portal, if this portal was placed appropriately during the diagnostic arthroscopy. The angle of anchor insertion must be from lateral to medial to avoid protrusion of the anchor tip at the subchondral level of the glenoid.

Most authors recommend anterior and posterior suture fixation of the unstable biceps origin. One double-loaded suture anchor under the biceps origin (or two single-loaded anchors) can be used. Normal variants of the anterior-superior labrum, such as a sublabral foramen (normal opening from 1 o'clock to 3 o'clock on a right shoulder) or "Buford complex," should not be repaired because this could lead to overtightening of the capsulolabral complex and postoperative stiffness, especially in external rotation with the arm at the side.[16]

Arthroscopic knot-tying techniques are critical with any arthroscopic repair technique (**Figure 5**). SLAP repairs differ from rotator cuff repairs in that the angle for knot tying is not always in line with the anchor. For posterior anchors, a cannula is often not placed through the rotator cuff, and knot tying is performed through an anterior portal. Many sliding locking knots require compression and reduction of the lesion with a knot pusher rather than with past-point tightening. However, posterior SLAP lesions cannot be effectively reduced from the anterior portal using a knot pusher. Therefore, sliding knots that use past-point compression techniques are preferred for obtaining adequate tension on the posterior portion of the labral repair. Alternatively, a small cannula can be placed through the muscle-tendon junction of the rotator cuff via the portal of Wilmington. This allows reproduction of the angle of anchor insertion for knot-tying utilization.

Case Management and Outcome Summary

This patient had a SLAP lesion that did not heal anterior to the biceps origin, with continuation of the detachment posteriorly to the 10 o'clock position. The drive-through sign was positive. Diagnostic arthroscopy revealed that the suture anchor was well-seated, but the suture loop was loosened such that the anterior-superior labral tissue was unstable under the loop. The intra-articular portion of the biceps tendon was otherwise benign.

Arthroscopic revision SLAP repair was successful. After fixation, the entire superior labrum was secure during manipulation of the arm into overhead positions. The drive-through sign was normalized, and the rotator interval appeared normal. The standard postoperative SLAP repair protocol was used, with the patient under supervised physical therapy.

Strategies to Minimize Complications

The diagnosis of a SLAP lesion is a clinical one and is based on a thorough patient history, physical examination, and other diagnostic studies. Ongoing pain and dysfunction following SLAP repair requires reevaluation of each category. If other concomitant pathology is ruled out, then revision of the SLAP repair can provide predictable improvement. The correct surgical technique and compliance with a supervised rehabilitation program are paramount for a successful result.

References

1. Andrews JR, Kupferman SP, Dillman CJ: Labral tears in throwing and racquet sports. *Clin Sports Med* 1991;10:901-911.
2. Snyder SJ, Karzel RP, Del Pizzo W, Ferkel RD, Friedman MJ: SLAP lesions of the shoulder. *Arthroscopy* 1990;6:274-279.
3. Andrews JR, Carson WG Jr, McLeod WD: Glenoid labrum tears related to the long head of the biceps. *Am J Sports Med* 1985;12:337-341.
4. Kim SH, Ha KI, Kim SH, Choi HJ: Results of arthroscopic treatment of superior labral lesions. *J Bone Joint Surg Am* 2002;84:981-985.
5. Rhee YG, Lee DH, Lim CT: Unstable isolated SLAP lesion: Clinical presentation and outcome of arthroscopic fixation. *Arthroscopy* 2005;21:1099.
6. Altchek DW, Warren RF, Wickiewicz TL, Ortiz G: Arthroscopic labral debridement: A three-year follow-up study. *Am J Sports Med* 1992;20:702-706.
7. Burkhart SS, Morgan CD: The peel-back mechanism: Its role in producing and extending posterior type II SLAP lesions and its effect on SLAP repair rehabilitation. *Arthroscopy* 1998;14:637-640.
8. Burkhart SS: Superior labrum anterior and posterior lesions, in Norris TR (ed): *Orthopedic Knowledge Update: Shoulder and Elbow 2*. Rosemont, Illinois, American Academy of Orthopaedic Surgeons, 2002, 543-549.
9. O'Brien SJ, Pagnani MJ, Fealy S, McGlynn SR, Wilson JB: The active compression test: A new and effective test for diagnosing labral tears and acromioclavicular joint abnormality. *Am J Sports Med* 1998;26:610-613.
10. Jobe FW, Bradley JP: The diagnosis and nonoperative treatment of shoulder injuries in athletes. *Clin Sports Med* 1989;8:419-438.
11. Kim SH, Ha KI, Ahn JH, Kim SH, Choi HJ: Biceps load test II: A clinical test for SLAP lesions of the shoulder. *Arthroscopy* 2001;17:160-164.
12. McFarland EG, Kim TK, Savino RM: Clinical assessment of three common tests for superior labral anterior-posterior lesions. *Am J Sports Med* 2002;30:810-815.
13. Swaringen JC, Mell AG, Langenderfer J, LaScalza S, Hughes RE, Kuhn JE: Electromyographic analysis of physical examination tests for type II superior labrum anterior-posterior lesions. *J Shoulder Elbow Surg* 2006;15:576-579.
14. Reuss BL, Schwartzberg R, Zlatkin MB, Cooperman A, Dixon JR: Magnetic resonance imaging accuracy for the diagnosis of superior labrum anterior-posterior lesions in the community setting: Eighty-three arthroscopically confirmed cases. *J Shoulder Elbow Surg* 2006;15:580-585.
15. Cohen DB, Coleman S, Drakos MC, Allen AA, O'Brien SJ, Altchek DW, Warren RF: Outcomes of isolated type II SLAP lesions treated with arthroscopic fixation using a bioabsorbable tack. *Arthroscopy* 2006:22:136-142.
16. Rao AG, Kim TK, Chronopoulos E, McFarland EG: Anatomical variants in the anterosuperior aspect of the glenoid labrum. *J Bone Joint Surg Am* 2003;85:653-659.

Chapter 9

Stiffness After Arthroscopic Instability Repair

Douglas H. Murray, MD

Case Presentation

Case 1

A 19-year-old, right-handed baseball pitcher presented with right shoulder pain while throwing. He denied any specific trauma, noting that the pain developed gradually over the season. Physical examination revealed a positive relocation test, a positive O'Brien sign, and a slight loss of internal rotation in abduction compared with the left arm.

MRI of the shoulder showed a superior labral tear, undersurface partial-thickness tearing of the rotator cuff tendons, and anterior capsular redundancy. The patient was diagnosed with anterior microinstability of the shoulder with internal impingement. Nonsurgical management failed despite a 6-week period of rest, supervised physical therapy, and an interval throwing program.

Initial Surgery

Diagnostic arthroscopy revealed a superior labrum anterior to posterior (SLAP) tear (**Figure 1**), and arthroscopic SLAP repair was performed with thermal capsulorrhaphy of the anterior capsule. Anterior and posterior biceps-flanking bioabsorbable suture anchors were placed. Thermal striping was performed over the entire anterior capsule, from the labrum to the humeral insertion. The rotator cuff tear was superficial and was débrided. Inflow of irrigation fluid was through the camera cannula, and suction outflow was through the thermal probe only. At the end of the procedure, a pain pump catheter filled with bupivacaine was placed into the glenohumeral joint to assist in pain management for the first 3 days postoperatively.

Following surgery, the patient progressed well initially, without acute complications or difficulties. He underwent a gradual stretching program over a 3-month period and started resistive exercises at 6 weeks. After regaining full range of motion, he began a throwing program at 5 months postoperatively.

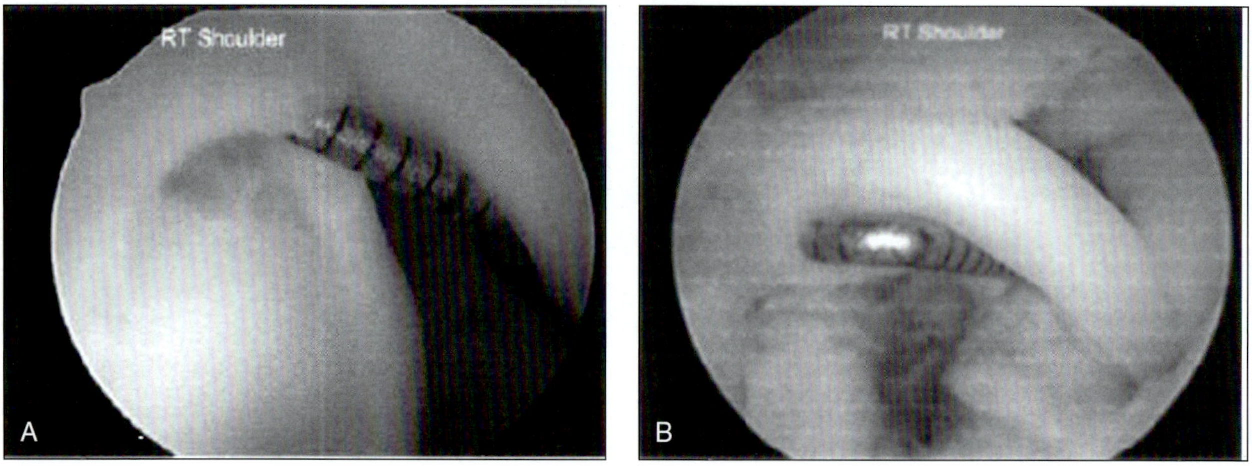

Figure 1 A, Documentation of the SLAP lesion. **B,** Repair of the lesion before application of thermal striping to the anterior capsule.

Current Problem

Seven months after surgery, the patient developed stiffness and pain in his right shoulder. His throwing program was stopped, but the pain persisted and eventually progressed to rest pain that was refractory to anti-inflammatory medications.

Repeat radiographs showed glenohumeral joint-space narrowing, with osteopenia and irregularity of the humeral head with subchondral sclerosis (**Figure 2**). An MRI scan showed a healed SLAP repair and stable anchor position, but arthritic changes were noted on the humeral head and glenoid surface. There were no lytic changes in the glenoid at the site of the suture anchors and no loose bodies.

CASE PRESENTATION

Case 2

A 28-year-old woman presented with recurrent subluxation in her right shoulder following a traumatic dislocation that occurred 5 years earlier. The injury happened when her arm was jerked by a rope while she was water skiing, resulting in an anterior dislocation.

The patient underwent closed reduction and began a supervised rehabilitation program that lasted for several months. Despite this treatment regimen, however, she had persistent instability and pain with overhead activities.

Physical examination revealed a bilateral grade 1+ sulcus sign, a positive anterior apprehension sign, a positive relocation maneuver, and a positive O'Brien sign. An MRI scan showed a type II SLAP lesion extending into an anteroinferior labral tear.

Initial Surgery

The patient underwent arthroscopic labral repair. The labral tear started at the 6 o'clock position and extended anteriorly up to the posterosuperior 11 o'clock position. The anteroinferior portion of the labrum was avulsed from the glenoid rim and had healed to the anterior glenoid neck. The anterosuperior glenoid rim was devoid of any labral tissue. The superior labrum was meniscoid in appearance, hypermobile, and extended directly into a thickened middle glenohumeral ligament (MGHL) (**Figure 3**).

Two anterior working portals were established, along with a posterior viewing portal. In addition, a transtendinous midlateral portal was created for placement of the posterosuperior suture anchor; the other suture anchors were inserted through the more lateral of the two anterior portals. Suture anchors were placed at the 5 o'clock, 3 o'clock, 1 o'clock, and 11 o'clock positions on the glenoid

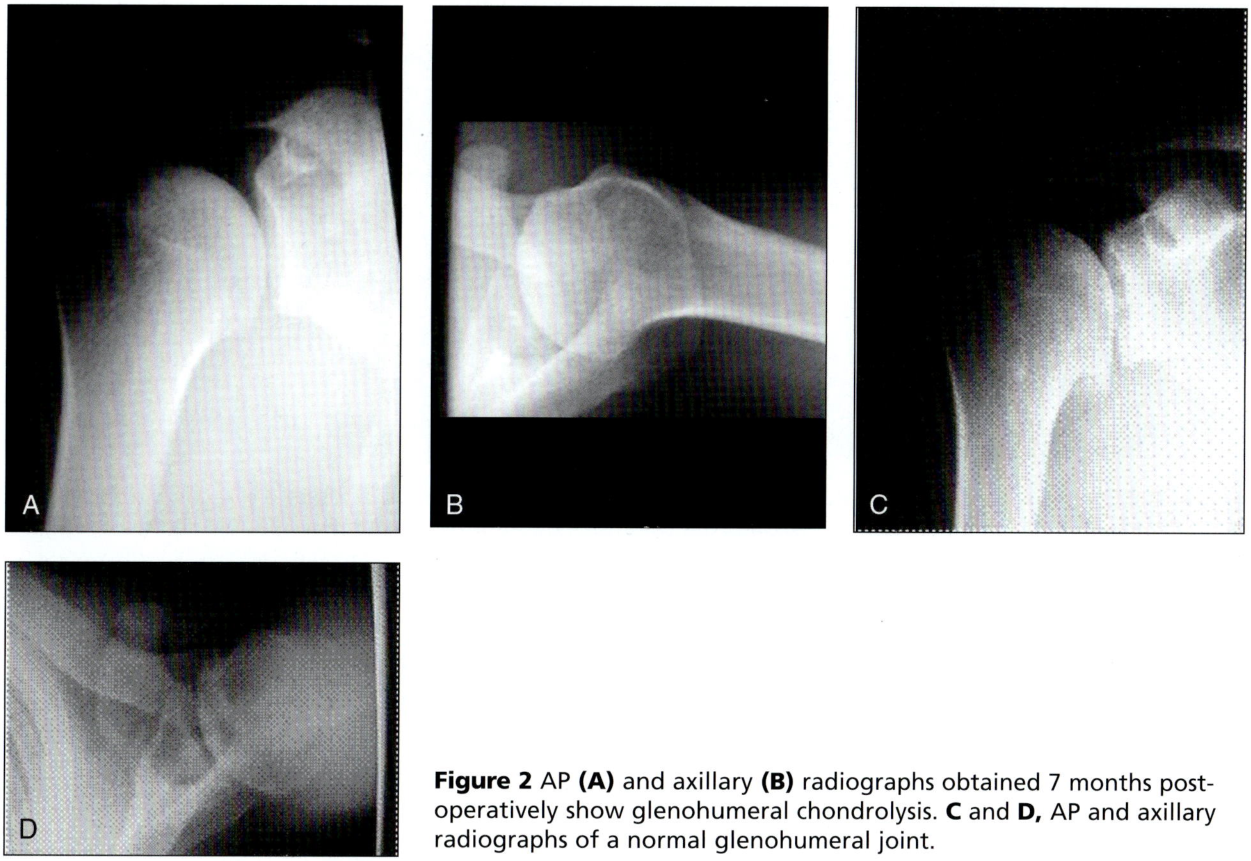

Figure 2 AP **(A)** and axillary **(B)** radiographs obtained 7 months postoperatively show glenohumeral chondrolysis. **C** and **D,** AP and axillary radiographs of a normal glenohumeral joint.

rim. Following repair, the entire glenoid rim was covered by labral tissue.

Postoperatively, the patient was immobilized in a sling for 3 weeks, after which active-assisted elevation was allowed up to 90° and external rotation was allowed to neutral. Six weeks after surgery, she was allowed to elevate her arm while internally rotated and to externally rotate while adducted, as tolerated; abduction with external rotation was avoided. By 3 months, she was still unable to advance beyond 10° of external rotation, despite home exercises and formal physical therapy. Forward elevation did not progress beyond 110°.

Current Problem

The patient had postoperative shoulder stiffness that had persisted since her arthroscopic instability repair. Radiographs showed no loss of joint space, and a repeat MRI scan revealed that the suture anchors were well positioned and the labral repair was intact.

A review of the arthroscopic images confirmed the repair of an anteroinferior labral tear and a type II SLAP lesion. Also noted was the preoperative labral configuration, which showed a cord-like MGHL complex with no labral tissue on the anterosuperior glenoid rim. This tissue was repaired to the glenoid rim with two anchors placed between the equator of the glenoid and the biceps origin.

Discussion

Shoulder stiffness after arthroscopic instability repair can be the result of many factors, including incorrect tensioning of the capsule or labrum, inadequate rehabilitation, or the development of arthritis in the glenohumeral joint. As with any

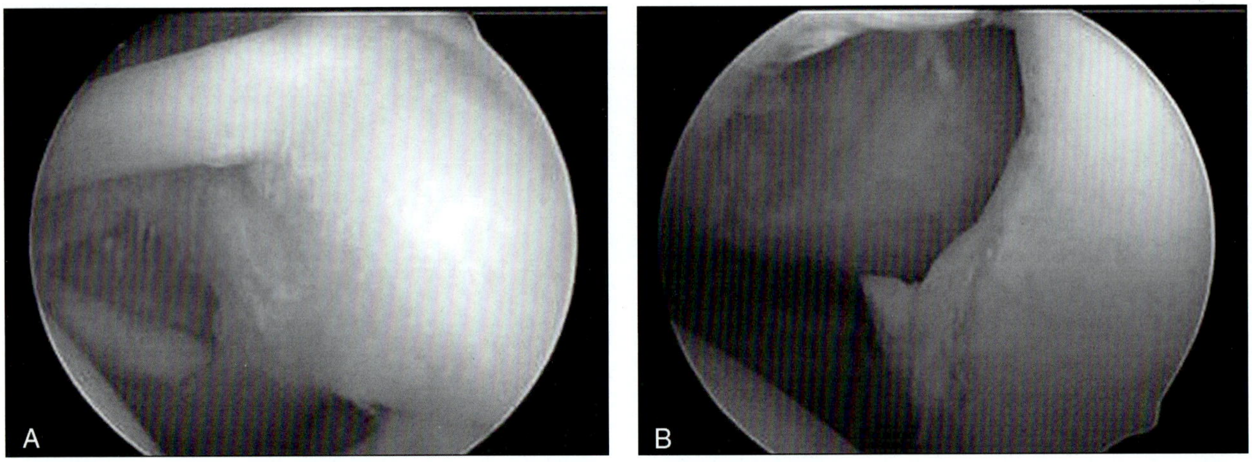

Figure 3 A, Arthroscopic image demonstrates the meniscoid superior labrum extending directly into a thickened MGHL. **B,** Arthroscopic images show that the superior quadrant of the anterior glenoid rim was devoid of labral tissue.

complication, the patient history is crucial for the evaluation of stiffness following instability surgery. The differential diagnosis is impacted by whether the stiffness persisted into the immediate postoperative period or developed after several months. Although rehabilitation regimens following shoulder instability repair vary, a near-complete return of motion is expected by 3 to 4 months postoperatively with steady patient compliance.

Recognizing and Managing Immediate Stiffness

Immediate stiffness may result from inadequate physical therapy, nonanatomic repair of the capsule, or mechanical problems caused by prominent suture anchors.

Inadequate Physical Therapy

Early stiffness should be treated aggressively with supervised physical therapy. Kim and associates[1] demonstrated that stable arthroscopic repair of the labral pathology will safely allow early rehabilitation of the shoulder. In their study, 62 patients with traumatic recurrent anterior shoulder instability underwent arthroscopic Bankart repair using suture anchors. One group of patients was managed with an accelerated rehabilitation program consisting of immediate postoperative staged range-of-motion and strengthening exercises. A second group was treated with 3 weeks of sling immobilization prior to initiation of conventional rehabilitation therapy. The patients who underwent early mobilization had a quicker return to a functional range of motion and a functional level of activity, without any increased risk of recurrent instability. With adequate therapy, full motion should be obtained by 4 months postoperatively.

Nonanatomic Capsular Repair

Nonanatomic repair of the capsule must be considered as the cause of stiffness if range of motion never reaches acceptable levels after shoulder instability surgery. Whereas historically, many open instability repairs were designed to be nonanatomic by deliberately overtightening the anterior structures of the shoulder, arthroscopic instability repairs can erroneously overtighten the capsule.

Typical Bankart lesions involve a capsular stretch as well as a labral lesion. An arthroscopically reconstructed capsulolabral complex can be undertensioned, leading to recurrent instability, or overtensioned, leading to stiffness. Accurate tensioning of the repair can be obtained by placing a temporary suture or by passing a grasper through the superior anterior cannula to hold the labrum reduced anatomically while suture relay is completed.

Reestablishing appropriate tension of the anterior band of the inferior glenohumeral ligament (IGHL) is the key to an anatomic repair. The damaged labral complex must be sufficiently released off the anterior glenoid neck all the way inferiorly to the 6 o'clock position to allow appropriate lateral and superior advancement of the prepared labral complex onto the glenoid rim. Suture anchors cannot be placed directly inferiorly on the glenoid; therefore, the released capsulolabral tissue is reduced by advancing the contiguous labral complex onto the more anterior suture anchors.

Nonanatomic repairs of normal labral variants can also lead to overtightening of the capsulolabral complex, with resulting loss of external rotation and forward elevation. The anterosuperior portion of the labrum has a range of normal anatomic configurations, which Rao and associates[2] observed in approximately 13% of shoulder arthroscopies (**Figure 4**). The surgeon must be able to differentiate these normal variants from pathologic lesions. One such variant is the presence of a sublabral foramen—a sulcus between the normally developed anterosuperior portion of the labrum and the glenoid articular surface. The sublabral foramen has been observed by itself or in conjunction with a cordlike MGHL complex. An absence of labral tissue on the anterosuperior glenoid rim has also been found in association with a cordlike MGHL complex.

The anterosuperior labral variations do not appear to contribute to shoulder laxity or instability. In Case 2, a Buford complex was "repaired," leading to excessive tightening of the MGHL and loss of external rotation. If nonanatomic repair of the anterosuperior labral variant to the glenoid rim is noted postoperatively by review of arthroscopic images and the surgical report, release of the incorrectly repaired tissue will be required to obtain full range of motion. This may involve simple suture removal or possibly arthroscopic capsular releases if the tissue has healed.

Prominent or Loose Suture Anchors

Early persistent stiffness with mechanical symptoms (pain, catching, and locking) may be caused by

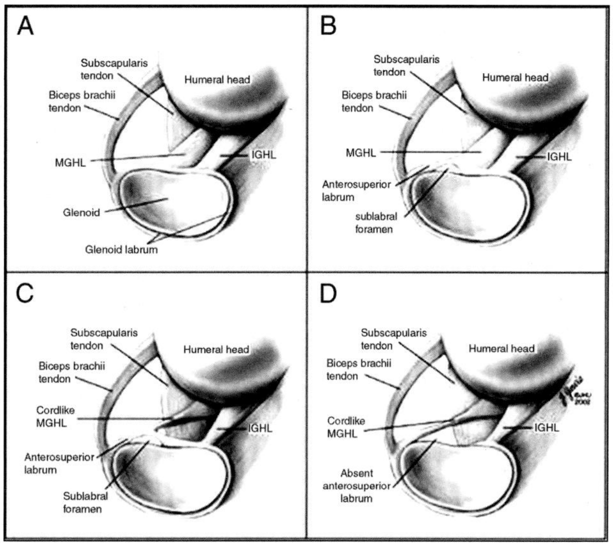

Figure 4 Normal anatomic variants of the anterosuperior labral complex. (*Reproduced with permission from Rao AG, Kim TK, Chronopoulos E, McFarland EG: Anatomical variants in the anterosuperior aspect of the glenoid labrum: A statistical analysis of seventy-three cases.* J Bone Joint Surg Am *2003;85:653-659.*)

prominent or loose suture anchors. Proper anchor positioning and purchase is critical to obtaining adequate fixation. To avoid shallow placement of suture anchors, arthroscopic portals must be placed sufficiently lateral to allow an adequate angle of anchor insertion into the glenoid rim. An anterolateral portal placed at the lateral apex of the rotator interval provides an adequate insertion angle for anterior anchors, and anterolateral and posterolateral portals placed 2 cm off the lateral acromion provide adequate insertion angles to the superior and posterior glenoid rims, respectively. The standard "soft spot" posterior portal and the central anterior rotator interval portal are too medial to allow a proper insertion angle; drilling and suture anchor insertion through these portals may result in shallow anchor placement and early loosening.

Adequate visualization is necessary to ensure that the suture anchors are completely seated and are not prominent. The use of bioabsorbable suture anchors creates a challenge in this evaluation postoperatively because these anchors are not well seen on radiographs. In such instances, a magnetic reso-

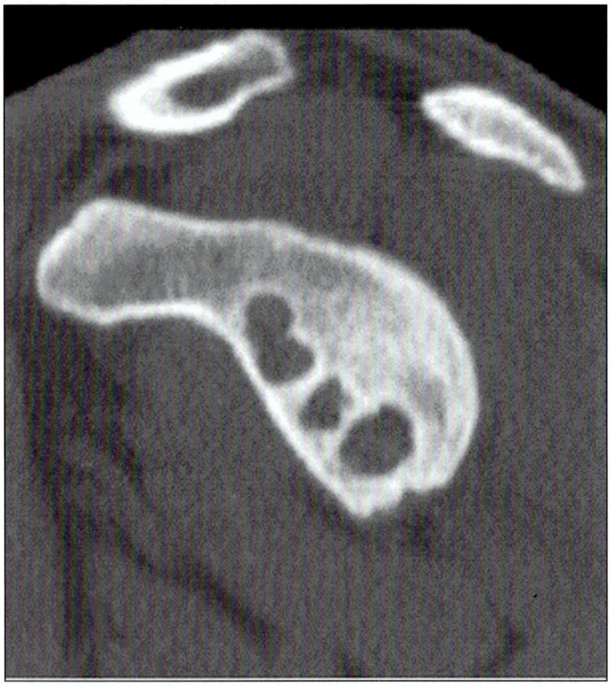

Figure 5 Coalescence of osteolytic lesions around absorbable suture anchors can lead to subacute anchor loosening. *(Reproduced with permission from Athwal GS, Shridharani SM, O'Driscoll SW: Osteolysis and arthropathy of the shoulder after use of bioabsorbable knotless suture anchors: A report of four cases.* J Bone Joint Surg Am *2006;88:1840-1845.)*

nance (MR) arthrogram or CT arthrogram can be obtained to look for foreign bodies or prominent anchors. Early detection with a high index of suspicion is required to avoid severe, permanent damage to the joint surface by loose suture anchors. Suture anchors that penetrate the articular surface must be removed immediately. Removing partially buried anchors can be technically challenging, and an arthrotomy may be required if the arthroscopic attempt fails.

Symptoms caused by prominent suture knots made of heavy, nonresorbable material are significantly less severe than those caused by prominent suture anchors and include irritation with a sensation of squeaking or even audible squeaking. This complication can be avoided by placing the post for arthroscopic knots on the soft-tissue side of the labral repair. The symptoms typically abate as the suture scars in with the capsule, but arthroscopic removal may be required if symptoms persist.

Recognizing and Managing Delayed Stiffness

Delayed-onset stiffness can result from synovitis, chondrolysis, or late loosening of hardware. A delayed loss of motion with pain typically represents an articular cartilage or synovial problem. Typically, this will become symptomatic by 6 to 8 months after surgery.

The etiology of delayed joint inflammation is likely multifactorial. Possible mechanisms include synovitis from the biodegradable suture anchors, late loosening of the anchors because of surrounding bone erosion, or chondrolysis caused by a mechanical or chemical irritant. Updated radiographs and possibly MR arthrograms are needed to evaluate the patient if range of motion and pain worsen postoperatively after a period of improvement.

Synovitis From Suture Anchors

Any type of suture anchor can cause an inflammatory response in the shoulder. Similar rates of asymptomatic cystic changes in the glenoid have been reported for shoulder repairs using bioabsorbable and nonabsorbable suture anchors,[3] and both polyglycolic acid and poly-L-lactic acid suture anchors have been shown to cause inflammatory reactions.[4-7] The inflammatory response caused by suture anchor absorption can lead to large osseous cavities that can coalesce, which may allow the anchors to loosen and become symptomatic after the labrum has healed[6] (**Figure 5**). A synovial inflammatory response has been reported in association with intact bioabsorbable anchors in up to 18% of patients.[7]

Upon presentation, the patient with delayed-onset stiffness must be evaluated as if there were an infection to rule out late septic arthritis. Blood tests and joint aspiration analysis, as well as updated radiographs and an MR arthrogram may help to determine the diagnosis. Synovitis can be managed effectively with arthroscopic débridement; if a full-thickness chondral defect is present as well, the results are not as predictable.[7]

Chondrolysis

Chondrolysis following shoulder arthroscopy was initially attributed, based on case reports, to damage caused by direct contact of a thermal probe with the cartilage, or indirectly from heating of the lavage fluid. Other possible sources of chondrolysis have now been identified; thus, the etiology of chondral damage may be multifactorial rather than solely related to the use of thermal devices. In addition to direct and indirect thermal damage, chemical toxicity from an intra-articular infusion of bupivacaine and mechanical trauma from anchors or instrumentation have been implicated as possible etiologies for postarthroscopic chondrolysis.[8-10]

In patients with chondrolysis, radiographs will show joint-space narrowing and subchondral irregularities (**see Figure 2**). MRI may be able to differentiate between synovitis and irreversible chondrolysis. Early detection is important because débridement of the synovitis has produced better results than any option for established chondrolysis in the young patient.

In many of the case reports documenting chondrolysis following arthroscopic instability repair or capsular release, thermal capsulorrhaphy was performed with a bipolar radiofrequency probe.[8,9,11] The heat of the thermal probe and the temperature of the joint fluid can be challenging to maintain within a safe range; therefore, if thermal treatment in the shoulder is used, the surgeon must be aware of appropriate fluid management techniques to minimize the risk of overheating the lavage fluid. Increasing the rate of lavage fluid exchange in the joint is accomplished by increasing the inflow and outflow through suction. Pausing or lavaging the joint between applications of heat also may help avoid overheating. In Case 1, the flow rate was slow, which may have allowed the joint fluid to reach unacceptably high temperatures and contribute to the chondrolysis seen.

In some reports, thermal chondroplasty has been promoted for patients with arthritis. Other authors, however, have documented chondrocyte death with this amount of heat; therefore, direct contact of the thermal probe with the cartilaginous surface should be avoided.

Another variable that has been reported as a possible source of chondrolysis is the placement of an intra-articular bupivacaine pain pump.[12] In vitro studies have demonstrated that bupivacaine is cytotoxic to bovine articular chondrocytes after less than 30 minutes of exposure,[10] and in vivo studies on rabbits have shown that intra-articular infusions of bupivacaine causes histopathologic and metabolic changes in chondrocytes.[13] Chondrolysis has not been reported in other joints when a postoperative pain pump has been used. Nevertheless, if a pain pump is used postoperatively, subacromial placement may be preferred over an intra-articular location until more research is done.

Case Management and Outcome Summary

Case 1

The patient developed chondrolysis 7 months after shoulder arthroscopy after a period of adequate progress. Because of his mechanical symptoms, lack of response to rest, and diagnostic study findings, an arthroscopic débridement was performed. No loose bodies were noted, and the superior labrum appeared healed. There were significant cartilage defects on both articular surfaces, and a chondroplasty was performed. Postoperatively his symptoms did not change dramatically, and the pain and stiffness persisted.

Because of the persistent symptoms and failure of arthroscopic débridement, the patient elected to proceed with humeral head resurfacing arthroplasty (**Figure 6**). Postoperatively, his pain improved with daily activities, but his motion did not progress beyond 140° of forward elevation and 30° of external rotation.

Case 2

The patient had postoperative shoulder stiffness following revision arthroscopic instability repair, despite appropriate rehabilitation. Examination under anesthesia showed elevation to 120°, and external rotation was limited to 10° in adduction.

Diagnostic arthroscopy showed that the labral tissues had healed to the glenoid throughout the arc of repair, and no loose suture anchors were noted. Arthroscopic capsular releases were performed selec-

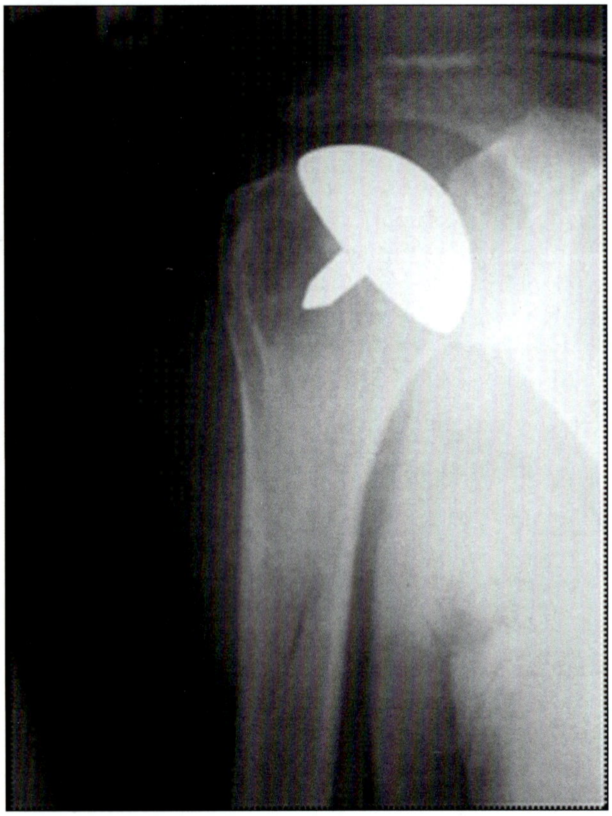

Figure 6 Humeral head resurfacing for chondrolysis of the humeral head.

tively just beyond the capsulolabral junction anteriorly, and the MGHL was released. The biceps origin and the anterior band of the IGHL were left secured.

Following the releases, the patient's intra-operative motion improved to 160° of forward elevation and 60° of external rotation. Postoperatively, she was allowed to increase her range of motion as tolerated. Two months after the revision procedure, she had regained the intra-operative motion, and her pain was significantly improved.

Strategies to Minimize Complications

Stiffness after arthroscopic instability repair can occur immediately or with a delayed presentation. A thorough review of the surgical technique, surgical pathology, and rehabilitation course is the initial step. Infection must also be ruled out. A careful history and physical examination, in addition to diagnostic studies that include radiography and possibly MR or CT arthrography, will be necessary to identify the source of pathology. In most patients, a successful recovery can be accomplished with early, aggressive treatment. Unfortunately, there are few promising solutions for the young patient with severe chondrolysis.

References

1. Kim SH, Ha KI, Jung MW, Lim MS, Kim YM, Park JH: Accelerated rehabilitation after arthroscopic Bankart repair for selected cases: A prospective randomized clinical study. *Arthroscopy* 2003;19:722-731.
2. Rao AG, Kim TK, Chronopoulos E, McFarland EG: Anatomical variants in the anterosuperior aspect of the glenoid labrum: A statistical analysis of seventy-three cases. *J Bone Joint Surg Am* 2003;85:653-659.
3. Ejerhed L, Kartus J, Funck E, Köhler K, Semert N, Karlsson J: A clinical and radiographic comparison of absorbable and non-absorbable suture anchors in open shoulder stabilization. *Knee Surg Sports Traumatol Arthrosc* 2000;8:349-355.
4. Edwards DJ, Hoy G, Saies AD, Hayes MG: Adverse reactions to an absorbable shoulder fixation device. *J Shoulder Elbow Surg* 1994;3:230-233.
5. Burkhart A, Imhoff AB, Roscher E: Foreign-body reaction to the bioabsorbable Suretac device. *Arthroscopy* 2000;16:91-95.
6. Athwal GS, Shridharani SM, O'Driscoll SW: Osteolysis and arthropathy of the shoulder after use of bioabsorbable knotless suture anchors: A report of four cases. *J Bone Joint Surg Am* 2006;88:1840-1845.
7. Freehill MQ, Harms DJ, Huber SM, Atlihan D, Buss DD: Poly-L-lactic acid tack synovitis after arthroscopic stabilization of the shoulder. *Am J Sports Med* 2003;31:643-647.
8. Levine WN, Clark AM, D'Allesandro DF, Yamaguchi K: Chondrolysis following arthroscopic thermal capsulorrhaphy to treat shoulder instability: A report of two cases. *J Bone Joint Surg Am* 2005;87:616-621.
9. Ciccone WJ, Weinstein DM, Elias JJ: Glenohumeral chondrolysis following thermal capsulorraphy. *Orthopedics* 2007;30:158-160.

10. Chu CR, Izzo NJ, Papas NE, Fu FH: In vitro exposure to 0.5% bupivacaine is cytotoxic to bovine articular chondrocytes. *Arthroscopy* 2006;22:693-699.
11. Jerosch J, Aldawoudy AM: Chondrolysis of the glenohumeral joint following arthroscopic capsular release of adhesive capsulitis: A case report. *Knee Surg Sports Traumatol Arthrosc* 2007;15:292-294.
12. Petty DH, Jazrawi LM, Estrada LS, Andrews JR: Glenohumeral chondrolysis after shoulder arthroscopy: Case reports and review of the literature. *Am J Sports Med* 2004;32:509-515.
13. Gomoll AH, Kang RW, Williams JM, Bach BR, Cole BJ: Chondrolysis after continuous intra-articular bupivacaine infusion: An experimental model investigating chondrotoxicity in the rabbit shoulder. *Arthroscopy* 2006;22:813-819.

Index

Page numbers with *f* indicate figures
Page numbers with *t* indicate tables

A

T

V

W